Born in Cyprus in 1947, George came to London in the mid-1950s. George's life experiences have been extensive and unique; working in the tourism industry, in photography and in building construction, he is now a successful singer.

George has had his share of 'ups and downs' but, whatever life has thrown at him, George has always maintained his beliefs in family values and enjoying life and has helped others to do likewise.

This book wasn't planned. It was inspired! It's written with George's heartfelt wish to assist others and to have a laugh along the way.

I would like to dedicate this book to humanity for the good it may bring for the journey ahead.

George Michaelides

DEPRESSION GETS LIFE AND GOOD RIDDANCE!

AUSTIN MACAULEY PUBLISHERS®

LONDON • CAMBRIDGE • NEW YORK • SHARJAH

A CIP catalogue record for this title is available from the British Library.

ISBN 9781035836482 (Paperback)
ISBN 9781035836499 (ePub e-book)

www.austinmacauley.com

First Published 2024
Austin Macauley Publishers Ltd®
1 Canada Square
Canary Wharf
London
E14 5AA

20241114

I would like to thank my wife Androulla for her patience, support, love and contribution which was most of what makes up Chapter 7 – the Good Stuff 2. Also, a big thanks for proofing, reading and typing the manuscript. Thank you to my mother, Theano, my brother-in-law Costas and my sister Thelma who gave me so much inspiration for just simply being a part of my life and their unexpected contribution whilst writing this book. Lastly, thank you to the publishers who believed in the contents of this book and went with it.

Table of Contents

Introduction

I started writing this Book in March 2022 and, as you can see, and probably might be a little confused about, is that the first chapter is entitled 'A simple guide to beating depression'. That's what it was supposed to be; a simple guide consisting only of just one chapter to be made available as an A6 pocketbook or an information leaflet. The title was changed more appropriately to the present one on the front of this book to reflect on the additional contents here, which resulted from circumstances and incredible events that took place from the time I started writing until the end. This subsequently added a further 13 more chapters on the subject. Events so surreal, so unexpected, that I felt compelled to carry on because it was necessary and appropriate; although sometimes painful but mostly enjoyable. What came out of me was documenting what was going on at the time, how it made me feel, and, even more amazing, it was spontaneous. My hand with a pen in it just kept on moving…writing…

I am happy that I did continue because what transpired was real, surreal and, although slightly contradictory in places, it was what was happening as I was writing at the time. What made it even more interesting, after I had written about something days earlier, 'lo and behold'! A front-page headline or inside article would appear in the newspapers actually commenting on one of those same subjects. Crazy or what? I just could not pass on that or pass on other unbelievable events which I felt should be highlighted for the good.

As I continued, I felt new personal experiences, new feelings that had no ending and new information about the subjects I was writing about coming in on a daily basis. I am happy to report that I did find the ending although I had my doubts. The ending was not far from what I believed and what I was writing about in the first place. Can you imagine that after writing a whole book, you discover that you were wrong because of the events now happening and because of new information coming in? Wow! That would have been awful! But, I guess the fact that you are reading this now, proves that what I have written about was indeed good and correct.

This book **is** about depression; the causes, the 'causers' and how to keep depression at bay and well away from you and me. There are thousands of books written which include pages on the subject and books just all about the subject. I have read a few of these books in the past and a couple during this writing. I have found, especially recently, that most authors, well-known scholars and past philosophers all agree on the power of the mind. The importance of how to control thoughts and how to use thinking to heal, react and use wisely for a happier and healthier life. I am very pleased about this because **the H.A.H.A. (Happy Achievement Happy Account)** concept described in this book, created by me ('pat on the back') is a simple and effective method adding to the many other self-help methods already out there. I say 'simple' because my book and method is easy to read and understand. This is unlike most books where you need a dictionary to look up every other word, and, where you are dazzled by endless scientific terminology. These types of books, written by all types of scholars, are great for scholars of all types, but are not so helpful among us non scholars; probably the greater majority of the population. I am therefore very pleased that this book can be read and understood by everybody.

I started writing this because I believed in a concept which I discovered the hard way by falling into depression and, finding a way out of that dark and horrible place that I was in, with experiences and answers that made sense and were proven to work.

The way you interpret thoughts; both consciously and unconsciously, together with a healthy diet and lifestyle, is most definitely the way to go or, as the Americans say, "You are good to go." What we have to acknowledge and, this is very important to note, is that our stress levels of everything around us, being the main cause of depression is now about ten times more than ten years ago and probably twelve times more; made worse by the Covid pandemic and other factors. Oh yes! Be aware of that.

This is why I have written about major contributors here in this book. These are actual stories and factual events that were happening as we came to the end of 2022. I wrote about these happenings for many reasons.

(1) To inform you that, even though we have found answers to being healthier and wiser, the opposition, the 'enemy', the darkness has been

getting stronger. It has infiltrated sections of our society we once depended on for customer care and most importantly the service for our health and wellbeing. Be aware especially if you fall in to depression and you cannot understand why. Know your enemy.

(2) To document these events as they happen for future realisation and teaching; unbelievable as they might seem.

(3) For selfish reasons; wanting to get these negatives out of my being so that I could make room for more positive and healthy thoughts.

(4) To urge Society that what we have endured in the last decade; especially in the last three years is unacceptable and changes must be made. This needs to start with the way the people who are paid to manage our affairs and our country do it right. Failure and waste should not be tolerated.

"When the going gets tough, the tough get going" as they say. Yes, the enemy is getting stronger, yes our stress levels have trebled. '*So,*' I thought, '*how can we fight back?*' I thought well, since we are putting this book together, how about some extra reinforcement? The UK at the moment, at the end of 2022, is in one terrible state as documented in this book. We cannot do much about that as it is mostly related to Government leadership and bad management. We therefore have to do the best we can and, again, just hope it is put right one day. The NHS is in dire straits which means our health is in jeopardy. This we can do something about while 'they' try and put this right too.

Bad health is a major friend of depression and so a good target for us to attack. Me and the missus therefore decided to include information in this book to help possibly to stave off decease and, if that is too late for some people, to help stop it from getting worse at the very least. I have to mention that there are no guarantees and to always consult your doctor if unsure about your decisions and health concerns. We have therefore written 'Chapter 7 The Good Stuff 2'. In that chapter, you will find information on how some parts of the body work, nutritional advice for health and an army of goodies at your disposal when the nasties come calling. Go in peace and in good health.

Chapter 1
A Simple Guide to Beating Depression – March 2022

Hello! Thank you for picking up this simple guide. Let me say right off that I am not a medical professional, social worker, therapist or any kind of holistic guru. I am a professional singer who has 'been around the block' a few times. I started singing in 2005 when I went into a small recording studio in Kentish Town, North London to record a couple of songs for fun and, realised to my amazement and, that of the people there, that I had a talent for singing! Since then, I have recorded two 12-track albums of covers, completed many, many, live shows and still perform when requested; pubs, clubs, private functions and so on…I have high hopes for my singing career so if you have some time, check me out at www.georgeides.co.uk. "**George Ides**" is my stage name by the way.

Singing – as is well-known – does have a healing effect on people and other living beings so I guess I am some kind of well man practitioner after all! Before the singing, I was a building contractor for quite a while, picking up the relevant qualifications along the way – through practice and at evening college – including plumbing, electrics, plastering, decorating and carpentry. Way before my building career and, after leaving secondary modern school – or more like being thrown out at the age of fifteen with no qualifications because that's what they did in those days – I entered the world of employment. Another thing they did in those days was that you were sent to see a careers' officer in school to help you on your way. The careers' officer asked me what I would like to do as a job and I replied, a photographer, please. In response to my reply, I was sent to work in a clothing making factory in Islington, North London! Another thing they did in those days, ignore you!

After a year there, I decided it was not for me so I got a job in the travel industry. Starting as an office junior and ending up as a freelance business travel consultant with Thomas Cook. I was also once a photographer, mini cab driver and a shop assistant in a grocery shop. I lived in Toronto, Canada for a couple of years and for a while drove one of those yellow taxis you see in movies. I also travelled quite a bit during my travel industry days, which included working for Egypt Airlines, Swiss Air as well as working for myself. I told you I had 'been around the block' a few times!

I will be 75 this July 2022 and am looking forward to what comes next; especially with my singing career and performing on the big stage. I did have an opportunity once to audition for Britain's Got Talent (BGT). I was approached and told to come along, avoiding stages one and two and onto stage three with the 'cameras rolling'. Unfortunately, I had a wedding booked for that date and could not make it. I did ask BGT for another day but was refused and so I missed an opportunity. I am sure there will be other occasions if you believe in yourself as I certainly do. Expecting me to cancel a wedding booking made months ago was not fair or realistic.

Writing about depression was my way to help to heal myself when I eventually discovered and accepted that I was suffering from depression. So, I thought, *If I am going to do this, why not do it in a way so that other people might benefit as well?* They do say that, if you do have problems, write them down as an initial step and go from there. Find the cause and rectify the situation. Easier said than done. But, it *can* be done. I have done it for myself and it has improved my life.

I am not saying it will improve your life as we are all different, but, there is a good chance that it *could*. I am not saying it will cure all, but it *might*. What I am saying, with confidence, it does help a lot and there are no medications or costs involved!

I lived with my lovely wife for over 30 years in Notting Hill, West London. Wonderful Kensington, down Kensington Park Road towards Westbourne Grove to Westbourne Park Road, just around the corner from Elgin Crescent Village by Portobello Road. Before my lovely lady came into my life, I was already a resident of the area having lived in several other locations for about twenty years. Having spent a life-time in Notting Hill, which I loved so much and having the privilege to meet so many people and become friends, including many market stall traders, the time came in February 2021 to make a move.

It was several years prior to our move when I realised I was suffering from depression. However I was not entirely sure what that meant and how it had manifested itself...During this dark period, we had problems with our neighbours with issues relating to noise, hygiene, drug abuse and anti-social behaviour. Living on the first floor of a house with four other flats and sharing the communal parts became a big problem. We were getting older and the other 'in and out' tenants were younger than us and less concerned about decency and respect. I suppose in the natural law of change, it was time to move on; especially when living in such a lively, young and vibrant area. Although, at the time, it felt more as though we were being forced out.

The fight for justice to assert our right to live in peace in our home went on for far too long. Being let down by people and organisations whom we trusted; whose job it was to support us − the good, the right, the law abiding − rather than abandon us; as they did, resulted in huge disappointment. A huge 'reality check' that led to, what I now know, to have been depression.

When I say people and organisations, I mean the police who 'turned their backs' on drug abuse, harassment and promises. Landlords who broke the Tenants' Agreements and also 'turned their backs' on prostitution, anti-social behaviour, drug abuse and health & safety issues. Our local authorities and MP who were sympathetic and, who promised action but, who chose, in the end, to forget about the problems or that we ever existed. Lastly, the Housing Ombudsman who is as effective as a campfire in the monsoon.

All of these huge disappointments and realisations came at a time when a very special uncle of mine passed away. They all took their toll on me. Things were so bad that I actually went to A&E at Charing Cross Hospital in West London and asked them to help me. My head felt heavy and wanted to drop off my shoulders, my eyes were blurred and wanted to close. I felt dizzy, tired and emotional; all of which are typical symptoms of depression as I now know.

I was examined by a lovely female doctor and I was surprised that I was not told to go away and take a couple of paracetamols. This doctor took an interest though and carried out several tests; all of which thankfully came back negative. So there was nothing wrong. However the doctor did notice that, a week earlier, I had been in the same hospital for a CT scan on my lungs as I was previously diagnosed for a possible problem due to scarring − found through an Xray I had prior to the CT scan − that showed signs of possible emphysema. Although when I was told about this originally, I did feel worried but I had actually forgotten about it with everything else going on in my life! It was, however, a contributory factor to the way I felt; like an ingredient to the depression, I now realise.

The doctor found the CT scan episode on my records and, being a great doctor, who obviously thought that this worry might be a contributing factor to my state of mind, told me she would get the results straightaway and come back. There were a lot of worries on my plate as she might have realised, so, if she were able to eliminate one, it would be a step forward. It would be great if every doctor were like this one; taking an interest and caring instead of trying to get rid of you with some suggestion or medication. The doctor came back and happily told me that there was a slight trace of the disease but certainly nothing to worry about! Nothing else showed up and I could leave.

It seems obvious, that deep down, I was petrified that I was doomed with this killer disease on top of everything else. Her words: "There is nothing to worry about" – those lovely words felt like a huge weight just fell off me and I generally felt well again; **like magic**.

I thought to myself as I was leaving the hospital – *Now with an appetite that I did not have before – heading to the nearest cafe, how can one bold action looking for help and a few comforting words change the situation?* After months of nothing but negative words, sad situations and responses. I realised then that there **is** a way in determining the way you feel. There is a way of combating and even beating, what I now know was depression. Positive action; looking for answers and a positive thought system.

Positive actions are easy to achieve. You just do it like I did! Look for answers and do not stop until you have a clear view of the problem. Meet it head on and 'nip it in the bud'. Do not fester on things. Sort it! Solve it! Move on! Happy, positive thoughts are not so easy to come by and I don't mean getting an ice cream or booking a holiday. These thoughts and actions are good but depression needs a **much** stronger opponent. Genuine kindness, generosity and respect towards yourself and to other people; with a strong, realistic approach to whatever comes your way – no matter how surreal – because surreal happenings are fast becoming a way of life it seems. **These are top gun opponents**.

Now, armed with this new realisation of events and my newly discovered wisdom, me and my wife decided to 'choose our battles' if not eliminate our battles altogether! We moved to Folkestone in Kent to live by the sea. It's much quieter and greener than Notting Hill and we have a flat in a solid block with neighbours of a similar age to us. A place where, hopefully, we do not have to rely on anything or anyone for support, which, as we had clearly found out during our time in London, did not exist as it was supposed to.

Although a big chunk of stress was eliminated in our lives, I still had to deal with the cultural difference. The move had a huge impact on me. After 50 years in bustling Notting Hill in the centre of London compared to the total opposite here in Folkestone, it has taken time to adjust However, now living here in Folkestone, I can say – with confidence – that depression in my life has been 85% eliminated, working on the last 15%!

Stress **has** to be controlled, reduced, erased and detached from your life as much as possible. If you don't like something, get rid of it or change it! Stay away from negative people and situations. If it means moving home, do it. Natural stress like losing one's loved ones, failure, being let down, failure in the system can be controlled and halted in time by creating a **H.A.H.A…Happy Achievement Happy Account**. Something to read about later here, with instructions!

Life will throw a lot of stress, anxiety and fear your way; that is inevitable. Death of loved ones and pets, family disputes, not getting what you have worked for, injustice…and it goes on! Politics, pandemics, wars, threats on your lives and it still goes on!

The result is depression, 'the Blues', 'down in the dumps' and lots of other descriptions. All in all, no matter how you describe it, it's **depression.** Yesterday, 15 March 2022 as war rages in the Russian invasion of Ukraine recently and after two years of the COVID pandemic, it was reported that mental health services in the UK recorded 4.3 million referrals in 2021 (and rising) as the disease continues to take its toll on our wellbeing. Pre-Pandemic recorded referrals were 3.7 million.

Sad reading indeed. Doom and gloom with no end in sight. To add to all of this – and including the war – we have been advised that our fuel bills, gas and electricity will be rising by up to 100% from April this year. Yes, there's no typing error – 100% – and this is in addition to practically everything else such as food, petrol, rents going up and it goes on! Ahhhh! Are you kidding? Is this for real? HELP! True, I'm afraid. Surreal!

More than ever therefore, as mere mortals we have to find ways to protect our wellbeing and sanity, by any and all means possible and available to us. Because the consequences are very bad news. There is not a lot we can do about the mess the world is in, we can only hope that the people who *can* do something, get it right.

"God grant me the serenity to accept the things I cannot change, the courage to change the things I can, and the wisdom to know the difference."

(Reinhold Niebuhr)

We all know about wonderful moments, winning money, new-born babies, the fun of pets, business success, good exam results and so on. But what we are looking for is more, more deeper personal achievements and good deeds.

It seems to me that depression is always there; lingering, standing by even though you have succeeded in financial goals, immediate targets and are comfortable in many ways. Or, if you are young, full of energy and have no time to be affected by it or even know it exists or what it is. Depression will hold you to account though as you get older if you are hit by circumstances that ignite it. I was hit in my late sixties because of circumstances mentioned before, although not as bad as it could have been because most of what I am writing about here to combat depression, I had already put in place naturally. When I refer to circumstances, I mean things like huge disappointments, unexpected stressful situations and bad health. Big triggers indeed. There's no need to go into any more detail about my misfortunes as this book is more about dealing with depression.

There are lots of 'wrong ways' in dealing with depression including:

1. Eating everything in sight; comfort eating for which there are lots of temptations out there; in fact everywhere you go.
2. Drinking too much alcohol.
3. Not taking any interest in social activities or exercises.
4. Smoking and using drugs.
5. Negative and vindictive thinking.

None of these activities will ever defeat depression. They merely feed it; causing obesity, looking older, loss of stamina, all kinds of health problems, more severe depression and, probably, an early death.

And now the Good Stuff

In order to reduce depression and, even beat it, you have to give yourself lots of Feel-Good Factors and Achievements; promoting happy positive thoughts when you need those most. Remember my good news from the wonderful hospital doctor. You have to build a mental **Happy Achievement, Happy Account H.A.H.A!** Something to dip into when needed and, just like money, the more you have, the more you can depend on. Having loads of money however, expensive cars, clothing and houses do not guarantee happiness or a depression-free life. Having a H.A.H.A, I believe, almost certainly will be a great asset and ally to achieving just that.

Happy Achievement, Happy Account H.A.H.A!

Deposits:

1) Looking after yourself, being aware of what a good diet is, knowing what is bad and good for you and never closing your mind to new developments, ideas and information.
2) Being respectful to yourself and other people. Being kind, generous and compassionate.
3) Knowing what a good weight is for you and achieving that weight.
4) Exercising regularly to your capabilities and being pro-active and less reactive.
5) Staying active socially and learning about ways to move forward positively to relieve anxiety, tension, headaches and achieving goals.

What is the difference between these statements for self-healing?

1) I am trying to achieve my desired weight.
2) I have achieved by desired weight.

1) I have to be more respectful to myself and other people; kinder, generous and compassionate.
2) I am respectful to myself and other people; kinder, generous and compassionate.

1) I have to get out there and achieve my goals.

2) I have achieved my goals, or I have today put in place actions to help me achieve my goals.

You will have more chance of glorious relief from depression if you go with No.2. Even with all of these positives in going with No.2, depression can be so severe at times, with no explanation as to why or to the cause but dipping into your H.A.H.A. will certainly help.

Holistic Remedies:

Yes, I am in favour of these natural products. I believe that natural workings of the body can be lacking in certain aspects which pure remedies might put right. A sort of 'reset' function effect on the body. Products like Bach Flowers and homeopathy; anything that comes from natural resources, can't be bad. I have personally used Bach Flowers and can say, with confidence, that my experience was positive.

There are many books on these products and practices, so check them out. As always, please consult your doctor if you have doubts or medical problems.

Counselling and Therapy:

Talking to someone about depression and your problems is always great; helpful and certainly soothing. A friend or partner; again, always a good thing. A professional practitioner if you can afford it. Mental health problems, as I mentioned earlier, are at critical levels now with backlogs on our NHS, along with other medical problems. Although great work is done by the NHS, the reality is that help could be a long time coming so self-help is crucial. H.A.H.A. will help. GOOD LUCK TO YOU. YOU ARE NOT ALONE AND IT'S NOT YOUR FAULT.

'To travel is to learn – To learn is to understand – To understand is to see for yourself'.

(George Michaelides)

This is something I wrote when I was selling travel seats. I have always wanted to put it somewhere and this spot seemed appropriate. Besides, travel is excellent for wellbeing.

As you carry on reading, I would just like to say that, after I wrote this – the first chapter – I found these words along the way which confirm my views and are like the H.A.H.A. method; an effective way to live your life. The words below also reiterate that stress, in all its forms, dished out especially by the very people we depend on for health and safety, needs to be eliminated and not tolerated, because 'they' are literally making us sick.

Here are the words:

"The long-term effects of stress hormones can push genetic buttons and create disease. Stress is when brain and body are knocked out of homeostasis, and it's the body's stress response that innately returns the body to balance. To live in stress is to live in a constant state of emergency mode for extended periods of time, which depletes the body's natural healing resources. All organisms in nature can tolerate short term stress, but when we are under constant stress, the response is turned on and we can't turn it off. Now we're headed for disease. Simply said if we are using all our body's vital energy for some threat-real or imagined-in our outer world, there is no energy in our inner world for growth and repairs. Your thoughts can literally make you sick. This is a solid example of the mind-body connection. It begs to question. If your thoughts can make you sick, is it possible that your thoughts can make you well? You will learn in this book that the answer is yes."

(Ref: Heal by Kelly Noonan Gores)

A wonderful book by Kelly Noonan Gores. I might also add however that you will learn from this book that the answer is also yes!

Chapter 2
Anti-Depressants

22 July 2022

I actually finished writing, when today, I noticed this article which came up on my mobile phone alerts.

Wednesday 20 July 2022. *The Guardian.*
"Little evidence that Chemical Imbalance causes depression, UCL scientists find."

Antidepressants used for low Serotonin levels, widely believed to be a main cause of depression, have come into question after a major review, found NO CLEAR EVIDENCE that low Serotonin is the cause. The report also states one in six adults and 2% of teenagers in England are now being prescribed with the supposed antidepressant drug and rising which is known to have severe side effects if stopped.

Other studies looked at the effects of stressful life events and found that the more stressful life events a person had experienced, the more likely they were to be depressed, showing the importance of external events.

Now 'that's a turn-up for the book' literally! Which goes to show that what I had discovered and wrote about here is actually a positive and accurate way to beat depression and I am so pleased about that. Talk about timing!

Again! "The more stressful life events a person had experienced, the more likely they were to be depressed."

When I took myself to A&E that day, I was:

1) Waiting for results about a deadly disease;
2) Was having trouble with nasty and abusive neighbours;
3) My close uncle had died on the day and;
4) People whose job it was to support and help us; because that is what they were paid to do, had abandoned us.

Talk about pressure and stress!

What I wrote here in this book before *The Guardian* report was published proves to be correct. It is bad enough having one problem to deal with, let alone four at the same time; as was the case with my experience. Meet a problem head on, accept it, 'nip it in the bud', sort it, solve it and move on. Natural stresses in life such as losing loved ones, failure, missing out on BGT, going thin on top, together with any other nasty stress, can be dealt with effectively with a H.A.H.A. Open your H.A.H.A. today. Stay one step ahead, be well!

Have I finished now? I hope so! Now back to the singing and The Royal Albert Hall? The Palladium? Your Wedding, Grandpa's or Grandma's 80th Birthday party? The village hall? Anyone? It's all good! Haha!

Chapter 3
Depression from Illness
24 August 2022

Stressful situations are one of the main causes of depression.

These can then lead onto poor diet, ignorance and negligence on how to maintain wellness. I have chosen this area of concern because it is an area which we could all do something about. Stress indeed is right up there as a major ingredient of most serious illnesses, including cancer and heart disease; two of the biggest killers in our world.

A lot of people carry on in their lives doing, eating and drinking what they want, ignoring symptoms that could be a sign of something sinister going on in their bodies. They could be lucky enough to live to a 'ripe old age'. This might be so in those far-reaching areas of the planet where people live a healthy life in not-so-polluted lands, who eat lots of vegetables and fruits and work their bodies. However, in the fast moving, polluted, benefits-easy jam packed, stress laced cities, the chances are not so great. Early death is a definite possibility. Fighting an illness with regular follow-up appointments and taking a whole load of pills every day must be daunting. Even worse, fighting an illness and being homebound with regular visits by medical staff and carers and having to take a whole load of pills must surely be even more daunting! I am talking about those people generally below the age of 80. People over the age of 80 might be in this situation but, because of their age, it's more accepted as a possibility. Those unfortunate people who have to endure these two types of living and, there must be millions and millions out there, cannot really escape depression, even if they are lovely, optimistic and happy people. The drugs, with the horrible side-effects, will soon douse those positives. Yes, of course, there are people who develop these nasty diseases even though they have lived a healthy life, but, we also know that it could have been through genetics. These are rare occurrences, however, compared to the masses who ignored and remained ignorant of the facts and signs until it is too late.

Depression is rife among these unfortunate people in our society. The fact of the matter though, depression is also rife among their families and close friends. Yes, that is a sad fact I am afraid. It is okay to say: "I have only one life and so I will enjoy it"; I am sure you have heard these words somewhere along the way, but their family and friends are not enjoying it. They suffer as well! My sister Thelma used to say those words when I would tell her to: "Cut the smoking, watch what you eat, do a bit of exercise, look after yourself please!"

Alas, even though she is younger than me by three years, she is homebound and lives her life as described earlier. Families who have a person like my sister and, although understand those words will, nevertheless, get depressed when they are there witnessing the decline and deterioration in health of their loved ones. Right before their very eyes and helpless to do anything about it.

I heard once that there was a top oncologist consultant specialising in lung cancer whose young brother died due to smoking; his specialist area and he could not save him. That must have been really hard for the consultant. Depression is a formidable enemy indeed.

These situations happen a lot and I am sure you probably know of someone, like my sister, if you do not already have someone in your own family. I hope not! You give the love, the kindness, understanding and respect, but it is also imperative for **you** to have somewhere to go for support. That is where developing a H.A.H.A. can help; especially if you deposit acts of support, understanding, love, being there at the end of the phone and showing respect and kindness to that person.

Having lived in wealthy, 'prim and proper' Notting Hill for so many years where there was a high standard of education, knowledge of society and healthy affluent lifestyles, I now realise – after moving to not so wealthy Folkestone – that there are lots of people here with obesity and health problems. In fact, it is very obvious. So the problem is still very much ongoing. I was quite surprised at the size of the problem in this part of the UK, taking into consideration how much information there is about health and diet out there. It seems more information is needed. So I am happy to be contributing with this book!

Depression can hit in many ways as is evident here in Folkestone. There have been many years of decline and neglect here which has had a massive downward impact on this once very affluent town with its wonderful huge red brick mansions everywhere; never mind the impact on the residents. Thankfully, Folkestone is enjoying a regeneration phase now with lots of new developments springing up to accommodate not only residential and educational needs but also new business opportunities. Things are looking up.

I have always been very alert and observant about health from a very young age. I would say around the age of twelve when I gave up my winkle pickers (pointed Rocker shoes) for trainers. I had a twin brother who was bigger and taller than me. It is said that when our mother gave us each a bottle of milk in our cots, on her return she would find my brother with both of them! My father in later years suggested that I follow a career in becoming a racing jockey. I don't know whether it was because he was a horse racing enthusiast and saw a potential somewhere, or because I was short! Motivated by being pushed around by my brother and at school because of my puniness, the prospect of riding a horse for a living and having my food stolen, I decided to fight back and so I took up jogging! I remember it so clearly because it was a momentous time in my life. Living at that time in Yonge Park Road, near Finsbury Park, North London, I jogged to Highbury Fields, did a couple of rounds and then headed back home. I don't know why I picked jogging but sixty-three years later, I am still doing it. I did not get pushed around anymore. I became bigger and taller than my brother and there was not a horse in sight!

The results from doing something about a problem and being successful has stayed with me up until today. **It works!** You **can** change anything, do anything. **YOU** have one life so it may as well be one where **you** have full control, enjoyment and opportunity.

Chapter 4
Medication – Friend or Foe?

Moving onto my later years, my over 60 years old period, I was told by a cardiologist who included a professor in the field, that I needed a pacemaker. Nothing to do with the pacemaker but, for other reasons, which I will explain later, I am supposed to be taking a 30 mg pill of Lansoprazole twice per day for the rest of my life. This was prescribed by my own doctor, and, in addition, I am also supposed to be taking 75 mg of aspirin once per day, 20 mg of Clopidogrel once per day and 80 mg of Atorvastatin (statin) once per day. These medications are also meant to be taken for the rest of my life as well as prescribed by another cardiologist for reasons explained later. The outcome is:

I did not have a pacemaker.

I do not take any of the drugs.

I have never been prescribed blood pressure pills.

Please however do NOT stop taking your medication or ignore advice from your doctors. We are all different and a great deal of effort and research on my part went into the choices I made about my health resulting in my decisions.

I have all the respect in the world for people in the medical profession, from nurses to surgeons, but, unlike a lot of people, I do not believe they are gods and that their word is final; far from it. You do not know what their beliefs are, their motives, how much they care about you, who you are or where you come from…

We know they are doing a job according to their experience and information that they have, but let's face it – how many times have you heard the words: "Oh, I don't seem to have that file on you" or "I haven't been sent that information on you"; scary stuff. Worse still, they never volunteer further explanation on your problem unless you are fortunate and have somebody who might. That would be rare. Diet related, exercise, alternative medicine, books to read, anything will do, but usually nothing. You can ask and I certainly would encourage that you always do, although don't get too excited, either your time is up or they simply do not know or care.

There are alternative ways and means, treatments and practices to take into consideration for most ailments if you are willing to research and look for them. In the following pages, I will illustrate the reasons I was prescribed the drugs I mentioned and the pacemaker. I will also describe the way we dealt with my wife's diagnosis of breast cancer fourteen years ago. Although my wife had all the necessary cancer treatment, I cannot imagine where we would be today if we hadn't done a lot of research and then made lifestyle changes. Indeed, I can't imagine where and what I would be if I had allowed the doctors to put a pacemaker in me and, if I had taken all those drugs prescribed for me. Thinking about it. I wonder how many people out there in similar circumstances to me and my wife did adhere to the norm, obeyed orders and just did nothing extra or questioned or looked for answers? '*Millions and millions,*' I would think. I have an example of a person we knew who followed only the doctor's advice, who did nothing; the example does not have a Happy Ending. More about this person later.

Taking drugs long term will probably have a detrimental effect on anybody. It is a given; not to mention the dreadful side-effects in the process. I was prescribed Lansoprazole because I had developed a vocal dysfunction to my singing voice. It was later discovered that I was suffering from acid reflux. Basically what this means, put simply, is that the acid with food contents goes backwards into the throat and mouth passing by the vocal cords and thus causing the damage. Therefore the drug is used to reduce acid and to line the stomach. Stopping the natural workings of the body is not exactly good news at any level to my mind and so I was not all that keen on doing that. I therefore decided to research the problem to try and find an alternative; anything was better than taking drugs for the rest of my life. I did do my research and yes, indeed, I did find alternatives and answers to the problem as listed below.

1) Get a one-inch-thick plank of wood. Place it under the legs of the bed at the headboard side so that the bed and your head – while laying down – are one inch higher than the lower side of the bed and feet. This will help in stopping any fluids going upwards returning back into the mouth; reflux

2) Reflux can be a serious problem if left untreated so, secondly, you have to train yourself to eat earlier, say before 6 pm if you go to bed around 10 pm. Ideally you need to give yourself four hours for digestion before going to bed. It wouldn't be a tragedy if you were to miss the odd hour from time to time or, if you have not eaten a lot, as long as it becomes a routine as part of your life for the future.

3) Do not overeat, especially in the evening. Avoid spicy foods, onions and garlic during this period again.

4) Avoid overconsumption of alcohol with or after food; again mostly in the evening. I say evening, in all cases because it is near to bedtime and in bed is where reflux normally occurs.

Problem solved!

As I mentioned earlier, I was prescribed statins, aspirin and Clopidogrel. The reason for these drugs was because during 2014 – eight years ago – while jogging, I noticed an ache in my right shoulder which seemed to be there consistently when I jogged. I mentioned this to my doctor and was sent to see a cardiologist. I had all the tests, and it was decided that I needed to have three stents inserted into the main artery to my heart. It had furred up and this was causing narrowing and a problem with blood flow. This is, of course, serious as a heart attack can happen. As a qualified plumber, I can understand this clearly because I know what can happen when pipes and U-bends get clogged up. They need to be cleaned out allowing waste water to flow out freely. I have cleaned out a few pipes in my time! A stent is a tiny spring like metal mechanism that is carefully inserted, using a thin cable all the way up to the artery via the wrist or groin area. When in place, they are opened up, stretching the artery walls and then released to stay there permanently. The thin cable is then pulled out. This procedure allows a free flow of blood to reach the heart once more. This surgery is all done whilst the patient is wide awake and also watching everything on a monitor.

After the three stents were in place, completed, at the Royal Brompton Hospital in South Kensington, London, the three drugs were prescribed, and the surgeon told me: "I'll see you in five years' time to do the other two arteries supplying blood to the heart."

I said, "Not if I can help it!"

Statins, as is well-known, are prescribed to be taken to keep these vital arteries from furring plaque known as cholesterol. Clopidogrel and aspirin are used to keep the blood thin for easier flow, especially at this crucial time after the stents were implanted. Taking these drugs forever was not something that appealed to me, but I understood it was important to obey; at least for the time being!

I was not surprised at my heart disease problem because, although I am generally conscious of my health now – being in my later years – I was not so concerned or, even knew much about the dangers of diet and lifestyle, when I left home at the age of 19 to share a flat with a couple of friends in Holland Park, Kensington, London. It was 1966, the famous '60s, buzz, buzz, buzz, the Beatles, the Rolling Stones, the World Cup, the takeaways, the smoking, the parties, the social drugs. Yes. I was there! I saw it, did it and, apparently, writing this Book about it! I therefore thought, *Taking these medications was certainly a good idea and I had no problem with doing just that.*

I carried on taking my medication religiously for about four years. During that time, I did make a lot of changes and improvements in my life. I educated myself to the facts on the problems I had which also included watching my diet, alcohol intake, upping my exercise routine and so on.

I did not go back for further stents after the five years as the surgeon had predicted. Instead, I stopped taking the statins. Statins do certainly work; my cholesterol main count went down from 6.0 to 3.5; even below the acceptable level of 4.0. The problem for me during the time I was taking the statins was depression; although I was unaware of what that entailed or knew the proper word for it. You hear people talking about extreme aches and pains as main side-effects; I would agree with that. The way I can be a bit clearer on this is simple. Basically if, like me, you have aches and pains beforehand due to probably the aging process; headaches sometimes, knee pain, neck aches and rheumatism, these ailments are heightened. They seem to go up a level, becoming worse when taking the statins. On further research into statins, I discovered that, if you have depression, statins can increase the level by 11% or, indeed, can start you on the road to depression which I personally believe to be true. No more of that! Thank you!

Aspirin and Clopidogrel promote blood thinning. This was obviously a necessary and important reason for me to take them after having had stents. However, after four years, with my improved lifestyle, I did stop these drugs as well, against the wishes of my cardiologist and my own doctor. Both these drugs can cause internal bleeding if not taken correctly individually. Taken together, as prescribed for me, can increase the risk of bleeding by up to 50%. Something I discovered through my research. I did not like those odds either individually or otherwise and certainly did not like what I read about taking them long-term. Bye bye little bleeders!

Again, please do not stop taking your medication. This is based on my experience and the way I choose to live my life. We are all different.

The Pacemaker Incident

In August 2016, I noticed by accident that I was developing a problem relating to irregular pulse beats. It was quite a weird experience. There you are, one day, sitting there and you decide to just check your pulse rhythm on your wrist as you do sometimes; well I do anyway…Expecting a nice smooth regular movement. Wow! What just happened? Who stole one of my pulse beats? Even scarier, then, I noticed two out of five of my pulse beats were missing. I waited a while and my pulse rhythm went back to normal but I knew where I would be going first thing in the morning, the doctors! I did go to the doctors and was sent for an ECG, Holter and pace treadmill tests at St Charles' Hospital, Ladbroke Grove, West London.

It all sounds very speedy as I write these events, but it took a couple of months for these tests to be completed. The only thing that was good in those days was that you could just walk into the doctors' surgery and be seen. Something that seems to have gone forever or so it seems for now, after the Covid pandemic. A doctor! What's that? Haven't seen one of those for years. Oops! Going off track here, back to the story.

One day while the investigations were going on, I noticed *three* missed pulse beats and then a *fourth* out of five. I felt sweaty and weak; maybe out of panic? But who would not be? Scared, I called an ambulance and was taken to St Mary's Hospital, Paddington, West London. I was there all day while tests were carried out. It seems I was experiencing something called ventricular ectopic heart beats. This is a type of arrhythmia or abnormal heart rhythm. It is caused by the electric signal in the heart, starting in a different place and travelling in a different way through the heart. This is not something I was told by the hospital doctors but something I learned about later after studying my own condition. What I was told at the hospital was: "Yes, we have done the tests and there is nothing to worry about, these things come and go, so you are free to go."

I questioned them because I was not happy with their casual report to something that did not exactly feel like 'nothing to worry about'. They said: "Okay, what we were looking for was something called atrial fibrillation. We are happy that it is not because this condition can cause you to have a heart attack or stroke. What you had was something similar that happens, will pass and not to worry, so you can go."

Happy that I did not have this atrial fibrillation disease, I thought I would heed their advice and get the hell out of there before they changed their minds!

I went back to St Charles Hospital for my follow-up appointment, now that the pain in the shoulder incident tests were complete. I met with a cardiologist consultant. He explained that, overall, they were happy with my results. I explained the episode at St Mary's Hospital and so the consultant wanted to carry out further tests. He also casually mentioned that, as a result of my missed pulse incidents, and their own analysis, I would probably require a PPM; also known as a pacemaker to be implanted in the near future. WHAT? I was sixty-nine years old. WHAT! He may as well have told me my life was over. That is the way my brain interpreted this information. Having a pacemaker fitted is a big deal as I knew it. Being told that I was the person who needed a pacemaker was an even a bigger deal! Talk about instant depression. Again, *WHAT?*

In fact, after carrying out my own research I learnt that, having a pacemaker does not change your life much apart from helping. You can pretty much carry on with your life and routine as normal. Nevertheless, a pacemaker! A contraption inserted into your body, attached to your heart! Horror! Horror!

I kept going back and forth to St Charles for about two years for tests and more tests and more consultations. In August 2018, I met with an arrhythmia nurse specialist who also told me that I needed a pacemaker and was ready to sign me up for one. Do these people get commission for signing people up? I felt as though I had been pressured; like the hard sell you hear about or like those people who try to sell you a timeshare or double-glazing.

During the past two years, I carried out a lot of research on topics relating to the heart and my studies led me to discover that my symptoms related to ventricular ectopic beats and there was a **cure!** Yes a cure for my condition! Although I carried on with my follow-up appointments, I was free from missed pulse beats for one and half years prior to the August 2018 appointment with the arrhythmia nurse.

By referring to the copies of medical letters and medical reports, I used the medical terms and words I found in them to carefully research their meanings online and in books. I stumbled on a report by Dr Sanjay Gupta on YouTube; a cardiologist based in York, UK. I have never met or spoken to this great man, but I hope to some day because he helped me cure myself! He introduced me to the **vagus nerve** and a cure for my missed pulse beats. Magnesium! It seems I was very deficient in this mineral and so I bought pumpkin seeds (rich in the stuff) and have been snacking on them ever since! The combination of stimulating the vagus nerve and intake of magnesium was my cure. Hey presto! No more missed pulse beats. THE VAGUS NERVE! What can I say about this vital hero in our bodies? Also known as the vagal nerves. These are the main nerves of your parasympathetic nervous system. This system controls specific body functions such as digestion, **heart rate** and the immune system. These body functions are involuntary; meaning you can't consciously control them. I will tell you more about the *vagus nerve* and Dr Sanjay Gupta later but, for now, I will continue on with the pacemaker saga.

On my appointment with the arrhythmia nurse, I told her about the magnesium and the wonders of the vagus nerve and therefore why I felt unconvinced that I needed the pacemaker. Up until this day I am still curious as to whether the nurse had even heard of the vagus nerve. Nevertheless, she remained firm in sticking a pacemaker in me. She told me she would arrange an appointment with a senior cardiologist to speak with me further.

On 5 November 2018, I met with one of the professor consultant cardiologists at St Charles Hospital. Wow! A professor. This was getting serious! He was adamant that I needed the pacemaker. I told him about the magnesium and the vagus nerve but he just shrugged his shoulders, ignored me and insisted he was the answer to my problem and he had the form to sign me up. I did not sign up because, as I told him, I was not convinced and intended to see what time would bring. He told me to be careful when driving or when up on ladders as there was the chance I could pass out, crash my car or fall off the ladder. Talk about hard sell! I was discharged. Eight years later, I haven't crashed my car or fallen off any ladders; not even close. I am free of missed pulse beats and my vagus nerve and I are on very good terms!

In April 2022, I instigated proceedings to have a check-up on the state of my old heart problem (bold action). I say instigated because, although having stent implants is quite a serious procedure, you do not get follow-up appointments to see whether further furring of the arteries has occurred. You also don't get to find out how the ones that were implanted are doing or even a: "How are you doing mate?"

I had noticed in the past year, periodically a slight numbness in my left arm. So I thought to report this and get that all important check-up in the process. It had been eight years since my procedure.

It worked! Later in the same month, I had an appointment with a cardiologist at the Royal Victoria Hospital here in Folkestone. In July, I had an echocardiogram stress test at Kent and Canterbury Hospital. This is some procedure! They put you to lay down on a contraption that is a horizontal iron bed with bicycle wheels. There you are laying down on this thing while the machine is manoeuvred in all kinds of directions, and you are peddling away. Your heart blood pressure is monitored while a person carries out an ultrasound to monitor your heart movement. A liquid substance is administered via a cannula, so that, as your heart rate increases, the liquid movement flow in the arteries is monitored for any potentially dangerous blockages. There is a doctor present ready to administer any necessary drug and to use probably any necessary equipment in case something goes wrong. In the meanwhile, you are encouraged to reach a heart rate of 125; this is helped by them making it harder to peddle, like riding up a hill. Quite an achievement to reach 125, when a normal heart rate is between 60-70. I did reach the 125 targeted heart rate and my torture was over, *phew*! My heart rate has just gone up recalling that experience.

A few weeks later, I got the report with the results from this test. The results indicated 'there was no inducible ischaemia. Ischaemia is a condition in which the blood flow (and thus oxygen) is restricted or reduced in a part of the body'. I was therefore discharged. I am happy that I investigated this procedure as I felt, taking into consideration the serious nature of my condition, it was important. Obviously 'the system' does not think likewise although heart problems are potentially life-threatening and the biggest killer in our society.

The last example regarding our medical problems was my wife's diagnosis of breast cancer. Yes it happened to us too. A huge blow and a major ingredient for depression. The horrible day was the 29 April 2008, fourteen years ago. My wife had had for many years a very lumpy left breast which often felt bruised.

But she wasn't worried because it wasn't a one-off pea-shape lump as we are often told and trained to look out for. Hers was nothing like that at all; more of an internal hardness that could be associated with various other conditions such as monthly cycles/periods. When she told me, I immediately told her to go and get checked out. She visited the doctor and was fast-tracked for an appointment at St Mary's Hospital in Paddington, West London. On the day she met with a nurse practitioner who examined her thoroughly. Unfortunately, the body language and comments the nurse made to two medical students who were present made it clear that things did not look good. A mammogram was arranged immediately, and my wife was told that she needed to wait and also see the consultant oncologist as she would need to have another test. Having done that, she was told to return later in the afternoon for results and yet a further test. Coming home to me alone must have been one of the loneliest and longest trips for her or any other human being to have experienced.

My wife came home and while I was working on the computer, she told me the news that we had to go back later. My world just came tumbling down, as I am sure hers, with all the interest directed towards her. We both sat down and stared at each other in shock, speechless with horrible 'What if' thoughts thumping in our heads.

The trip to the hospital in the afternoon with me and sitting in the hospital waiting area is embedded firmly in my mind, forever. As I write and recall the proceedings about one of the worst periods in both our lives, I find it hard but am happy that, by putting these experiences on paper, I will hopefully clear them from my insides; a bit like clearing a memory stick, and I can be assured that, once I finish recalling and writing this, I never have to do it again.

The words from the consultant as we sat in front of him were: "Yes, you have breast cancer."

(We later had the full diagnosis stage 3, grade 2 oestrogen positive). If I am talking about deposits in our H.A.H.A., this was the biggest withdrawal, bordering on bankruptcy. Absolutely devastated. We both went home holding each other and holding back the tears. When the trauma wore off a bit and we were able to speak, we decided to fight all the way.

The next horrible experience was to go back to St Mary's and to have various scans to determine whether the dreaded disease had already spread or not. Bluntly speaking, whether die or not. We waited for 10 days for the results. I stopped work from my building business to be fully hands-on to support my lovely wife. We just waited for what seemed to be forever and told nobody; just us two together in our worst nightmare.

On 9 May 2008, we were informed that the disease had not spread. So relieved! Our feelings were totally the opposite from that day when we were given the worse news of our lives. Good news indeed even though we were told that a mastectomy would be necessary and, to follow up with chemotherapy, radiotherapy and strong intensive medication (hormone therapy) for a long period of time. Horrible times ahead, but we were happy we had a chance. The mastectomy operation happened, the chemotherapy happened, the radiotherapy happened, and the loss of hair happened.

Truly a horrible, gruelling period in our lives and I witnessed the whole thing as I stuck by my wife all the way. To watch another human being fight for life and all those other people in the chemotherapy room; all sitting side by side while the chemo drugs were being administered, also fighting for their lives, was one of the most humbling experiences for me. In fact, some of the people in that line were actually dying in front of our eyes as it was too late for them, and they were given the treatment just to stay alive. All heroes in my eyes as was my wife – my main hero.

When the three main procedures were completed, my wife was prescribed a drug called Tamoxifen. In addition to all the previous horrible lifesaving experiences, the drug was no exception with terrible side effects including fatigue, hot and cold flushes, dreadful insomnia, night sweats, depression and aching joints. After three years, the drug was changed to a drug called Anastrozole, with less horrible side effects for a further seven years. Both hormone medications help reduce and stop any reoccurrence of the disease. In January 2019, the drugs were stopped after 10 years, and discharge was in March 2018.

My wife was already researching, reading and learning more and more about nutrition and complementary medicine way before her cancer showed up. These subjects were of great interest to her and also because she wanted to help close loved ones with their own medical problems. From the minute we were both told the disease had not spread, she went into overdrive to find ways and means to fight back. She got me involved and, I suppose this is where I got the experience in wanting to explore nutrition, to help myself in later years with my own medical problems. Funny thing about writing, you get to find out a lot of truths as you go along…I have a lot to thank my wife for, my hero. You also have to relive those times; good or bad and that can be difficult but gratifying to know it helps the writer and, hopefully those readers who get to learn and feel a genuine experience.

Talking about heroes, my wife was the most uncomplaining person during her illness and also can be thanked for all the hard work put into help complete this book. All of the information found in 'Chapter 7: The Good Stuff 2' is down to her. I think it would take another book to tell you about my special lady. But, for now I need to finish this one!

One of the first questions we were eager to ask our consultant oncologist who gave us the bad news – which we did – was: "What can we do to help ourselves fight back?"

His reply to our surprise and horror was: "NOTHING! Just carry on the way you are, as normal, we will do what is necessary."

We said, "What about food, drink, there must be something we can do?"

He again said, "Just carry on as normal."

The nurse specialist who supports patients was very kind but simply gave us a booklet on breast cancer; it had nothing on fighting back or nutrition.

We were hoping for a lot more positive advice; something, anything…alas, that did not happen. There was information on claiming benefits and what experiences to expect with treatment and so on…But nothing on fighting back.

We could not accept this advice to simply do nothing. There had to be something, anything to help fight back? There was! Foods, minerals and vitamins to consume, foods and other products to avoid and so on. The following pages and Chapter 7 The Good Stuff 2 is where you will find information on what we discovered, researched and put into practice. You will find ways to, not just do nothing, but to fight back and fight good!

What confirmed our actions to look for answers – years later – and not to just do nothing, to question, to delve and delve and not just take the word of a highly respected surgeon, was the fact that a friend of my wife's had also being diagnosed with similar breast cancer the year beforehand. This is the example I mentioned earlier on. A lovely lady who, unfortunately did 'do nothing'. She carried on as normal, making no big lifestyle changes or looking for ways to fight back. She was totally reliant on the care of her medical team, and she went into remission but, unfortunately her cancer returned twice. My wife tried to help her with what she had learnt. But unfortunately, it was too late and regrettably her friend passed away in 2019; three years after the second recurrence. 14 years later my wife is still with me. Whether it was the positive thinking, all the love for her, being active, the minerals and vitamins, the foods we introduced and the ones we gave up, who can say? However, we both firmly believe these actions were necessary and effective in our fight and, with thanks, I can write about them today.

"When the going gets tough, the tough get going." (Bold action).

As my wife's breast cancer was oestrogen positive, one of the first things we put into practice – as we discovered – was to stop all consumption of cow related foods; cheese, butter, milk and so on. Just a quick bit of information, although there are lots more to be found in Chapter 7 The Good Stuff 2. These diseases have a habit of often coming back, as we all very well know. So, anything you can do to keep them away so that you can have a happy and long life is very worthwhile, even if this means never going back to your old familiar lifestyle.

We carried out a lot of research on our conditions and paved the way for us to live our lives disease-free. We made choices and are happy that, it seems, these choices were correct with healthy and happy results. Bold actions; as mentioned before, look for answers and make the right choices for yourself. Medication is a bit trickier. They do work for millions of reasons but can also be very damaging if the problem is not fully investigated and understood. Sometimes research can provide alternatives that might be less damaging than conventional medication. Make sure you make the right choices and do consult your doctor first. He may not be God or have all the answers, but you need to know what the problem is first before you seek a second opinion.

Chapter 5
The Vagus Nerve

During my research looking for answers in the middle of my missed pulse crisis, I came across information on the vagus nerve. I had never heard of this nerve before and, by the reaction of many well-read people whom I mentioned it to, (including medical professionals), neither had they. Without being too scientific about this, I will try and keep this explanation simple, as I think sometimes that is the best way. I will tell you about this wonderful tool in our bodies and how to maintain it so that it maintains you; one of its many jobs. Being too scientific? I couldn't be even if I wanted to, I am not built that way. If you want more scientific stuff and, indeed more information which I do recommend, there are lots of books on the subject and there's always Dr Sanjay Gupta on YouTube.

Although not as famous as other nerves in the body, I am confident that you will be hearing more and more about the vagus nerve in the future. One book I came across was written by Maria Hampton entitled *Vagus Nerve Secrets – Your definitive guide to freedom from anxiety, depression, trauma, PTSD, inflammation and autoimmunity through self-healing techniques and exercises.* WOW! Sounds good! *Freedom from?* I think it is a bit optimistic, but to help in combating, managing and keeping depression at bay is definitely doable. The vagus nerve is the second longest nerve in your entire body; the first being the sciatic nerve. The vagus nerve is part of the body's nervous system; the term vagus means 'wandering' and that is precisely what it does. It runs through the entire body from the brain, reaching all the way down to the colon, touching on many systems on the way. The nerve also connects with organs such as the lungs, heart, intestines, stomach and bladder; to name but a few. Each side of the vagus nerve has up to 100,000 nerve fibres of which, 80% are sensory. It is an essential part of the immune system, sensing when and where there is inflammation in the body and helping to reduce it.

That is as scientific as I am going to get! So, we have this nerve with connections from the brain to all vital organs from top to bottom, literally. So, in theory, if something were amiss with one of these very important organs, the rest of the other organs will be affected as they are all linked. Moreover, however, something that hits home clearly, if there is a mental problem – anxiety, depression, the brain connection – you can say with confidence, that a whole load of negativity is going to reach all those vital parts. Stomach, loss of appetite; feeling sick, lungs; difficulty in breathing, heart palpitations, bladder problems and wanting to wee. So the way I look at it, if we want to be well, we have to control negativity and look after our vagus nerve as the transporter of vibrations to our bodies' working system.

The way the story goes is that the vagus nerve, with all its very important connections, needs constant stimulation so that it works positively, passing on goodwill vibrations everywhere. Some recommended practices for great stimulation of the vagus nerve include cold showers or, if you are like me, cold water over the head will do! Humming, singing, good digestion, diet and positive thinking. There are lots of more ways to stimulate this very important part of the body for good health so do investigate further! Get to know your vagus nerve, excellent for depression. There will be more information in Chapter 7 The Good Stuff 2.

'I have a feeling', a message to the brain via the gut, (gut feeling). 'You are getting on my nerves'; the vagus nerve is not happy. (You are bothering my vagus nerve, which, in-turn, bothers my other vital parts in my body).

Chapter 6
Surreal the New Real

So there are lots we can do to help us live a healthy, happy life. Not easy with surreal happenings now becoming the New Real. The latest news today 29 August 2022 is that the recent heatwave experienced in London and suburbs of up to 40° C, breaking all past records, is going to be the new norm. The forest fires this year mainly in France and California and other small ones experienced in lots of other countries are also something we are going to have to get used to as part of our lives in the summer periods. Pakistan was hit with severe flooding due to an extreme monsoon season in the last couple of days, killing thousands of people. Pandemics, threats of nuclear wars…We have experienced the unexpected; surreal the New Real.

There are many ways to be thrown into depression; more problems, failed relationships, failure in general and many other situations as mentioned before. One of the culprits which has become so clear; I would say especially in the past decade, has been the health service in the UK. I cannot comment on other countries but, here, it is very clear.

Our health, our families' health, our friends' health; it does not get any bigger than this. Most of the other causes can be worked on and put right, but our health involves putting our trust, our beliefs and our lives in the hands of other people and services. These same people; our Health Service, has made us fight to be seen and heard. We are lied to, abandoned and treated like idiots.

The Health Service, **what** health service? Since the Covid pandemic coming up to three years now, the Service has declined dramatically and, even though the pandemic has subsided considerably in the last year, the NHS has stayed in decline and has introduced a system of fight for your life for everyone. What I have experienced here is appalling and can say, as a fact, is probably causing the rise in mental health cases and onset of depression for many people. Thousands of people are dying daily because of delayed treatment or undiagnosed health problems. Dying before their time; surreal and very sad. What about their families? How do you cope with knowing your loved ones could have lived if the health service – which is supposed to be on top of things and trusted – let them down? I think I would probably be in depression for ever if I were one of those people. Words used such as unprecedented, blah, blah, blah! Governments across the world were warned of such disasters, medical and otherwise as I have discovered. Some heeded the warnings and so the impact was not as great, others, including the UK failed miserably.

Other services have also declined. We went through years of negative responses. Remember?

"Sorry your teeth have fallen out because of Covid." "Haven't managed to fix your car/fridge/bike/leak/boiler or your brain because of Covid." Can't answer the phone, return your email or 'give a toss' about your problem because of Covid. No one seems to mention Covid anymore but the services have still remained in decline.

Apart from all the unnecessary deaths and worsening of ailments people have to endure and the horrible consequences that they have to accept, I personally resent the way people are being treated, lied to and taken for idiots.

"This is a very busy time for contacting us. Please try again later."

It does not matter what time you call, it's the same message. Lie!

"This is a very busy time for contacting us. Please try later."

And then you are cut off. Rude, disrespectful and made to feel abandoned.

If you don't get cut off and have been sitting there for 30 minutes listening to the same crap recording over and over, go through all the options and still hanging on, you decide to 'cut your losses', keep your sanity, hang up and have nothing to do with this company again. If it's health-related, well…the fight goes on.

So! So far we have natural disasters getting worse year by year and meetings of promises of action by heads of governments happening frequently but we have yet to see any positive results.

We have a health service that is not working with the outcome of needless deaths, waiting lists for help that are hopeless including mental health. We have organisations where we are customers or patients, including the health service, that have resorted to blatantly lying to us, abandoning us and treating us like idiots.

To someone suffering from a mental health problem, as well as all the new cases which have arisen with all that has happened in recent years, the outcome has been depression. Abandonment, being lied to, being treated like an idiot, not being able to get crucial help when needed or at all. All these things just add 'fuel to the fire' which, inevitably, results in isolation, withdrawal, severe depression and, regretfully, sometimes suicide.

When we get ill, whichever form that takes, our 'first port of call' is to our doctor. I haven't seen a doctor ever since the pandemic; coming up to three years now. I have spoken to one a few times but even that was quite a mission. On one occasion that happened this year 2022, I spoke to a doctor and complained about periodic dizzy spells. He referred me for blood tests. Two weeks after the blood tests there was no news as to my results. I tried calling the surgery a few times but the task was a bit depressing as I couldn't get through on the phone. Three weeks went by; still no results. I had a physio appointment at the surgery so I decided to make enquiries when I was there. At my physio appointment, I asked the receptionist about my blood test results. She looked at my file and reported: "Oh yes, your tests came back normal." I asked why I was not informed and she said, "If tests come back normal, we do not respond."

News to me! Obviously I was happy that my blood tests – for what I do not know for – were normal. So, what's next? I still would like to know, facts and figures, an explanation or something. I still have periodic dizzy spells. For all I know, my problem has not been resolved, what next? The answer from the receptionist, "I don't know, I am not a doctor." Precisely! The doctor or assistant should speak to the patient. The receptionist agreed but, to do that, you have to make an appointment by calling again at the appropriate time 8am in the morning. Argghhh! Surreal! Frustrating! Annoying! Aren't surgeries supposed to make you feel well?

My surgery boasts that when you call, to save time, use a service on their website called an E-Consult available between 8-11 am. Sounds good! So, as I was still waiting to find out more about my periodic dizzy spells I decided it was important to have more tests and answers, even though the surgery did not really seem to care. The next day I got up early and was ready to try the E-Consult service, ready for the 8am kick-off. I logged onto the surgery's website where I am registered and at 8am, I got going. The process felt promising and I managed to fill in the questions which took about seven minutes. I pressed submit. Argghhh! The reply was, "This cannot be accepted, call the surgery."

Frustration! Anger! Abandonment! Aren't surgeries supposed to make you feel better? What is more annoying is that I had wasted ten minutes of my time which could have been used trying to get through on the telephone. I was now 33rd on the queue and, of course, by the time I got to one in the queue all the appointments had gone for that day.

The next day I got up early again and was ready to telephone promptly at 8 am. Two minutes into dialling and the line was busy with a recording saying, "Sorry all appointments for today have now been taken, call back tomorrow." How could that be? It was now only 8:02 am. Even if each call took five minutes to complete, it is impossible for all appointments to have been taken up in two minutes. Lies, lies, lies. Abandonment. Annoying. Regret. How can this be happening?

The very people whom we go to for help, support and for medicine actually cause a lot of our problems especially with regard to mental health, as what I have described here is literally messing with people's heads and, if people already have messed up heads. Well, you can see where this is going! The sad thing is that these practices cannot see the damage they are causing; treating people like beggars who are trying to get something for nothing, when, in fact, they have paid and are paying for these services.

I was frustrated with not being able to get through to my surgery and concerned about my wellbeing so I tried calling 111; the health service one down from the 999-emergency service.

The response was, "This is a particularly busy time for our service, maybe you can call back another time."

I hung on and listened to about 15 minutes of recordings about all kinds of stuff which consisted mostly about how to get rid of me, I eventually gave up after 15 minutes and hung up. A very sad state of affairs from a country supposed to be 'up there'. My advice to you is stay healthy because nobody knows how long this insanity is going to go on for. I still don't know what the cause of my dizzy spells were. I could have a brain tumour for all I know? I know one thing. Nobody but me seems to care. Thank God that I am not in a seriously depressed state or I would never recover. Some people however are seriously depressed. I feel for them having to endure such diabolical treatment from the very people they depend on for help and who, in reality, make things worse. This situation is happening now.

Talking about happening now, here's a real incident. My wife developed a nasty cough just after we came back from a disastrous trip to London on the 28 December 2022; you can read about this in later pages. We thought it was a cold and would soon pass so did nothing about it. By 9 January 2023, her symptoms seemed to be getting worryingly worse and so we decided to call 111 at about 1 am on the morning of the 10th. Oh, yes! There it is again: "This is particularly a busy period for us, call back later." It's **1:00am** in the morning! Needless to say that was a lie (what's new) as someone answered after five minutes. The call centre assistant went through endless questions with my wife after which she said, "A clinician will be calling you back within two hours."

We felt good as now we were doing something about the situation which had become a worry; especially taking into consideration my wife's past medical history. We stayed up all night waiting for that promised call which unfortunately did not happen. Lies and abandonment. Here we go again! At about 7am we called 111 yet again to find out what was going on. After the usual crap and further lies on the recording, a person answered after about seven minutes. My wife protested that the promise of a call within two hours never happened and she had sat up all night waiting for the call. The assistant apologised, although it seemed clear that this was not an isolated incident, more of general practice and he said that he would put a chase on the call.

As it was now approaching 8:00am and with the disappointment with 111, I had the idea to try and get through to our doctors' surgery. Armed with three phones, we left the one expecting the call from 111 and used the other two to call the surgery. We both called at the same time using the appointment line. Yes here it is at 8:02am.

"All the appointments for today have been taken, try again tomorrow."

Lie! I told my wife to just stay on the line. After listening to the usual crap trying to get rid of you, I was greeted with the message saying that I was seventh in the queue. Eureka! I was in. A few minutes later, my wife got the same message telling her that she was tenth in the queue. Phew! We were at least in the queue and phew two we would finally be able to get something sorted out. Now I actually had reached number one in the queue and my wife had reached number six. Things were looking up and I actually thought about telling my wife to hang up her phone, but something told me not to; a gut feeling. Bang! Suddenly, after sitting on number one for a while, I was cut off. I got cut off! After all we had gone through from 1 am until now, this now happened.

Take a bit of time and put yourself in our place, how does that feel? From someone who has experienced this there are no words; well at least no decent words. My wife was now number one in the queue. Please God don't let them cut her off as well! Now they got us praying for our health, sad! Eureka! She was answered; a live human voice was on the other end asking, "How may I help you?"

After the usual questions, my wife was referred to the local minor injuries unit at The Royal Victoria Hospital for a 10:50 am, checkup. Wonderful. A result! It turned out that my wife was suffering from laryngitis and a chest infection so we got the mediation and went home. On our return home, we discovered missed unknown calls. Two messages from 111. 10 hours later. Too little, too late.

Worries, followed by lies, abandonment, deceit, more lies, stress and depression. It really is amazing that there are people (in the health service in particular) who are paid to come up with ideas and problem-solving and, all they can come up with, are lies and deception undermining the intelligence of our society. You might come to expect it from other greedy organisations but not from an organisation that you have placed your trust in to help. Who are these people? Who and why is this allowed to carry on? Shame on you sad people, sad, sad, people.

The NHS was a great dream in its concept. A bit of a foolish dream in my opinion. They did not think about greed, corruption and fraud. If they did, it was okay because it was government owned so no individual could ever lose money. Only the country's finances lose. Politicians and people running it just kept pouring money into the service with all kinds of associated firms, people and organisations making huge amounts of profits from it; pocketing vast amounts of what was going in, leaving anything that was leftover for actual care and carers. It was never enough for care and, still as evident, not enough to keep doctors and nurses; some of whom opt out for private work paying bigger wages. Recently it was reported that £2 billion was spent in locum/temporary doctors and nursing staff in one year. With all this going on, things do not look promising in the future. In fact, nurses have voted to go on strike at the end of the year 2022 for the second time in their history. Waste, waste, waste. Doctors and nurses trained by the NHS only to leave and go to work for private medical employment agencies and assigned back to the NHS for double the money; crazy, crazy, surreal!

I have managed to look over some NHS guidelines: paperwork sent to those lucky people who have registered depressed with their doctors and managed to get a response. Most of what I read were great instructions and similar to what I have mentioned here in this book.

Keeping healthy, exercise, socialising, positive thinking and how you interpret thoughts. All good stuff. Furthermore the guidelines state:

Thoughts:

People who are depressed tend to think very negatively about themselves, the future and the world around them. It can be like seeing life through 'gloomy specs'.

1) Everything is hopeless – nothing can change.
2) I am useless, worthless.
3) It's all my fault.
4) The world is a terrible place, everything goes wrong.

As a person who has experienced depression, I can safely say I have never felt any of the itemised symptoms described here. I think maybe they should include five. Being let down by the very people who are supposed to be looking after them.

I agree some people do have these thoughts and feelings as itemised. People who have been brainwashed to believe that or have not looked for answers elsewhere or, in fact, people who are bordering on mental problems, paranoia or other serious mental issues. Sadly, they do see life with 'gloomy specs' and these people certainly do exist. All very sad, bless them.

There is however very little mention of the people who get depressed, some very seriously, but who still believe that everything is not hopeless, that things can change or improve with a bit of bold action, love and kindness and who speak up about, shout out loud about defects in the system. People who do not regard themselves as useless or worthless? Try getting up on a stage with hundreds of people watching and singing to them. That is not useless or worthless.

Some things can be our own fault, maybe little things but certainly, definitely not all our fault. The world is a wonderful place. Some things do go wrong, mostly things we can do nothing about, but certainly not a bad place.

People get depressed because, unlike successful results, positive responses, being respected and so on, things to be deposited into the H.A.H.A. (where it is possible to draw confidence and wellbeing from), we are bombarded by negativity on a daily basis. I am not talking about rude people in shops, people on buses and other situations in our everyday life. Yes, we can do without that because we know there are more good people than bad out there. And, besides, we can go weeks without encountering some turd with an attitude. What I am talking about is injustice, unfairness, obvious faults that people make excuses for, ignore and pretend are not happening. Major players like:

The Health Service.
The Police.
Government Departments.
Local Authorities.
Major product companies.
People who are paid to look after us and do their jobs, but do not.
Organisations which fail to deliver the results and services that we pay for.

Failure results in injustice, abandonment, disappointment, threats to your life, being ripped off and, when being obviously treated like idiots, lied to, disrespected, it all ends in depression. It's the old cliché.

"Blame it on greed" or "Blame it on the Government." Sounds about right!

I do apologise for bringing you down, as I feel down just writing these true factual disturbing statistics, but somebody has to.

Quick! What's in my H.A.H.A.? Oh yes, that feels better: Wrote ten pages today, went jogging this morning at the Leas Promenade, telephoned some old friends yesterday, I am in good health and going to stimulate my vagus nerve with a cold shower. Well, unlike my wife who can do that, I am just going to shower my head. A bit of a wimp me. Feel better already.

In the next chapter – The Good Stuff 2 – you will find information on foods, vitamins, practices and more information on nutrition as researched by us. This information and practices helped me and my wife with our medical misfortunes and we are happy to be here today to pass on the information. It is a guide that hopefully will be of interest to you, your family and friends. But, please read the information in the context of your own problem and/or condition and always consult your doctor if unsure.

Chapter 7
The Good Stuff 2

1. A strong and healthy immune system
2. Healthy bones
3. Maintaining stable blood sugar levels
4. Inflammation
5. Acidity in the body
6. Digestion, absorption and guts
7. The Brain
8. The Vagus Nerve
9. Ageing
10. Cancer
11. The Heart

1. A Strong and Healthy Immune System

A strong immune system is a strong fighting force and a defence against any disease.

A weak immune system is a warm welcome to any nasty forces.

1) Vitamin C is the 'backbone' of any immune-boosting system.
2) The brain communicates with the immune system cells all over the body.
3) The immune system cells communicate back to the brain using messenger cells (neuropeptides).
4) Each cell has a cellular memory!
5) **Everything** that strengthens our immune cells also hinders the growth of cancer cells; e.g. diet, exercise, stimulating the immune system, fighting inflammation etc.
6) Every few days, the body replaces a quarter of all its immune cells.
7) Stress hormones bind to immune cells, hampering their ability to fight illness by lowering the body's defences.
8) Laughter helps the immune cell receptors from binding to stress hormones.
9) Depression lowers oxygen levels in blood and cells by up to 30%. This helps cancer to thrive as it hates oxygen!
10) It's **not** enough to boost the immune system; also need to find ways to boost the white cells to help them recognize a cancer cell. (Vitamin D and Vitamin K help!)
11) Iron helps carry oxygen to all cells in the body including the immune system cells.
12) The body needs water – daily four pints/ two litres daily/ eight glasses…

If the immune system cells become dehydrated, the body draws water from bloodstream.

This makes the blood thicker and sludgier and makes the heart pump harder to push the blood cells around the body.

As the blood cells carry the oxygen around the body, this all causes tiredness and sluggishness.

The mucous membrane is one of the immune system's physical barriers.

Drinking water means that the mucous that coats your throat and contains antibodies, can trap cold viruses!

When the body doesn't produce enough mucous, viruses can survive better so drinking lots of water is essential.

The immune system has lots of different types of cells.

- White cells – leucocytes – form the natural defence against **all** rogue invaders.
- These white cells include T-Lymphocytes, B-Lymphocytes, Cytokines and Immunoglobulins.
- Phagocytes (neutrophils – 60%) and macrophages. Neutrophils swallow bacteria whole and live for approximately 36 hours before they have to be replaced.
- NK cells – Natural Killer Cells – 'special' white blood cells.
- Gut bacteria control approximately 85% of the immune system and up to 85% of our 'immune memory' is directed by the bacteria in our gut!

Note: Sugar inhibits phagocytosis; process by which viruses & bacteria are engulfed and literally chewed up by white blood cells!

Exercise is an immune system **booster.**

- Exercise helps white blood cells sweep back into circulation from where they are stuck on the blood vessel walls.
- Exercise reduces stress, it improves sleep, it changes the balance of hormones and it change the body's chemistry by improving its ability to remove sugar from the bloodstream.
- Exercise calms the mind and body as stress hormones are neutralised by endorphins.
- Exercise reduces the inflammation throughout the body.
- Exercise pumps your heart faster and this stimulates the thoracic duct; the largest lymph duct in the body. This allows the flow of white immune cells, energy flow etc.
- Exercise helps the heart become stronger as blood is more oxygenated.
- Deep breathing kick-starts the lymph system; clearing stagnant air from the lungs.

As with other body functions, diet is also important for the immune system. Boosters include: Fish oil, leafy greens, nuts and seeds, garlic, ginger, turmeric, citrus fruits, poultry, coloured vegetables, yogurt and olive oil.

2. Healthy Bones*

As we get older, our bones get weaker and are subject to easy breaking and possibly months in hospital so maintaining those bones is essential for a better life.

Bones are made of living tissues!

- An adult skeleton is made up of 206 bones.
- Blood cells grow in the bones.
- The body contains one kg of calcium. 99% inside your bones and teeth.
- The amount of calcium in bones is very carefully regulated by hormones.
- Oestrogen regulates the amount of calcium in the blood and slows bone loss. This changes after menopause when oestrogen levels drop.
- Our bones are continuously being replaced.
- Bone forming cells (osteoclasts) travel through the bone, in search of *old* bone. These osteoclasts eat away/dissolve the old existing bone that needs renewing and at the same time, release calcium into the bloodstream. This process leaves tiny unfilled spaces where osteoblasts move in.
- The osteoblasts build *new* bone and also deposit calcium into it.
- With age, the activity of osteoclasts and osteoblasts is no longer equal. The body loses more calcium than is put back and so bones lose density!
- Exercise stimulates bones to manufacture cells.
- It takes nearly 10 years to fully renew the skeleton, so an 80-year-old will have had eight versions of replaced skeleton!
- For most people, the answer is not boosting your calcium intake. The answer is how to reduce calcium loss.
- High acid foods cause calcium to leach from bones and be excreted in urine as well as reducing iron being absorbed. Examples of these foods include alcohol, caffeine, cheese, eggs, fizzy drinks, red meat, salt and sugar.
- Vitamin D helps our bodies absorb calcium. Vitamin D is synthesised by the action of sunlight on the cholesterol layer under our skin; so our body needs some exposure to sunlight.

- The body needs magnesium to efficiently absorb calcium, e.g. from oatmeal, potatoes, lentils, nuts and chickpeas.
- The body needs both Vitamin D and magnesium to get calcium out of the blood and into the bones!
- If over 50 years old, take calcium carbonate with meals; helps absorption. Calcium citrate is okay on empty stomach.
- Spinach, peanuts, rhubarb and sesame seeds contain phytic acid and oxalic acid. These block calcium absorption.

Foods 'rich' in calcium

- Calcium with Vitamin D helps absorption
- Almonds (contain trace mineral boron which helps prevent calcium loss and helps maintain Vitamin D in the body)
- Apricots (dried)
- Beans (baked, dried)
- Blackcurrants
- Berries – blackberries, raspberries
- Bread – good quality; wholemeal/organic/sourdough
- Broccoli (NB broccoli tips have more Vitamin K than the florets)
- Cheese
- Chickpeas
- Figs
- Fish – oily
- Hazelnuts (contain trace mineral boron which helps prevent calcium loss and helps maintain Vitamin D in the body)
- Hummus
- Kale
- Kiwis
- Mushrooms – one of the few dietary sources of Vitamin D
- Okra
- Parsley
- Pecans (contain magnesium) work with calcium to make bones strong
- Salmon, sardines, seaweed
- Seeds – pumpkin, sunflower

- Tahini
- Water (bottled)
- Watercress
- Yoghurt

* (Healthy bones include teeth)

3. Maintaining Stable Blood Sugar Levels

Out of control sugar levels – a nasty force to keep at bay. Diabetes is a growing problem.

- **ALL** sugars are converted into glucose.
- The body immediately releases insulin into the bloodstream to enable sugar/glucose to enter cells.
- Some glucose goes to the brain and muscles where it's used as an energy fuel.
- **ANY** excess glucose goes to the liver where it's turned into fat and stored.
- This fat storage causes weight gain. Insulin is known as 'the fat-storing' hormone.
- Poor insulin control is known to cause glucose excesses.
- Glucose excesses cause increases in oestrogen and inflammatory hormones throughout the body.
- Eating one large meal the day 'plays havoc' with insulin levels because the body becomes flooded with glucose.
- It is far better daily to eat 5-6 much smaller meals than one large meal, so…graze…
- Various factors affect blood oxygen levels including smoking and depression.
- The brain uses approximately 75% of all the glucose that circulates in the blood.
- The brain is absolutely dependent on a stable supply of blood sugar. Red blood cells are renewed every four months.
- Healthy cells break down a much smaller amount of glucose and breathe with oxygen (*aerobic*).

Cancer

Cancer cells get their energy and breathe differently to healthy cells. They break down unusually large amounts of glucose and breathe **without** oxygen (*anaerobic* respiration).

If cancer cells are starved of glucose, they cannot grow and divide.

Cancer cells take iron from the blood and that reduces the blood's oxygen carrying ability – hence tiredness.

High Glycaemic Index foods raise insulin levels and high insulin levels can contribute to cancer growth.

Glycaemic Load and Glycaemic Index

- Glycaemic **Load** is a unit of measurement that tells you exactly what a particular food will do to your blood sugar.
- Foods with High GL raise blood sugar levels in the body.
- Foods with Low GL help the body to burn fat.
- Glycaemic **Index** – tells you the ranking of carbohydrates from 0-100.
- This range 0-100 indicates how quickly food affects your blood sugar, i.e. whether it is fast (bad) or slow releasing (good).
- Blood sugar levels are affected by the presence of too much oestrogen!
- The hormones insulin, glucagon and adrenalin all control sugar levels.
- Refined sugar is a high GI food and anti-nutrient that increases insulin levels.
- The immediate rise of insulin is accompanied by the release of another molecule IGF-1 (Insulin-like Growth Factor).
- IGF-1's role is to stimulate cell growth; both insulin and IGF promote inflammation. Inflammation leads to a weakened immune system, cancer growth etc.
- Aim for low GI foods as they help regulate blood sugar levels and keep them stable.

To balance blood sugar

1) Eat less, eat better, eat often and eat good fats.
2) Avoid bad fats. Fats don't affect blood sugar but the amount and type of fat eaten will still affect your weight.
3) Eliminate/reduce allergies/inflammatory responses.
4) Exercise each day as muscle burns more energy than fat.
5) Exercise is the fastest way to improve your metabolic rate.
6) Exercise is the 'enemy' of cancer as cancer thrives in the presence of low oxygen!

GI foods

High levels of GI foods raise insulin levels which causes inflammation. Inflammation helps sustain growth of tumours.

If the tumour's environment is deprived of inflammatory factors needed for its growth, the tumour will **not** succeed in spreading. Therefore, aim for low GI foods.

These help to regulate blood sugar levels which, in turn, reduces insulin secretion which, in turn, reduces the growth of cancer cells.

Low GI foods

Foods that can reduce inflammation tend to be low GI foods. Examples include:

- Apples – Green apples have less sugar than red apples (approximately one teaspoon less)
- Beans
- Beetroots
- Berries: raspberries, blueberries, strawberries (contain more Vitamin C than oranges)
- Blackcurrants (weight for weight four times more than oranges)
- Carrots (contain chromium which can help stabilise blood sugar levels)
- Cherries
- Ginger
- Grains such as quinoa, bulgur and buckwheat
- Green tea – 200x more potent than Vitamin E and 500x more than Vitamin-C
- Kiwis (one kiwi has more Vitamin C than one orange)
- Lentils and pulses (also provide valuable protein)
- Linseeds/flaxseeds – the only 'seed' in the entire plant kingdom that contains three times more Omega 3 than Omega 6
- Mushrooms
- Nuts: almonds, walnuts (Note: nuts do NOT contain Vitamin B which is essential for cells)
- Oats
- Olive oil

- Oily fish – long chain: Fish that swim in cold water (e.g., tuna, rainbow trout, mackerel, salmon) keep warm by producing Omega 3 fatty acids. These block certain compounds that promote tumour growth.
- Parsley
- Pasta
- Pomegranate juice
- Rice
- Turmeric – most natural anti-inflammatory to date
- Unrefined foods

4. Inflammation

Inflammation is one of the nasty forces which we can certainly do without. A major nasty player.

Foods that are anti-inflammatory include:
- Beetroot
- Berries (raspberries have highest Zinc content of all fruit), Strawberries (help with absorption of iron and calcium)
- Brazil nuts (ideally in shells) for selenium
- Broccoli – tenderstems are crossed with kale and contain far more Vitamin A than normal broccoli; as well as C, K magnesium and potassium.
- Cabbage – red cabbage has 10x more Vitamin A for eye health and 2x more iron than greens
- Cherry juice
- Fish
- Garlic (red garlic has three times more allicin than white bulbs) – single best anti-cancer vegetable. Also contains tryptophan, the precursor of serotonin, the precursor of melatonin.
- Giblets
- Grapes (dark red contain resveratrol).
- Green tea (antioxidant)
- Kiwis (Vitamin C)
- Mangoes (antioxidant)
- Mushrooms
- Nuts – Brazil, pecans (Vitamin E), pine nuts, pistachios
- Oats
- Offal (selenium)
- Oranges (40% more Vitamin C in blood oranges than navel)
- Peaches
- Seeds – pumpkin, sunflower
- Shellfish
- Tomatoes
- Turmeric (antioxidant)

- Walnuts
- Watercress
- Watermelon
- Yoghurt (live/active)

Both insulin and IGF promote inflammation from the rise of blood sugar in the body.

1) Many cancers are directly linked to a chronic Inflammatory state.
2) Cellular inflammation drives cancer growth.
3) If cancer is deprived of the inflammatory factors needed for its growth, it will NOT succeed in spreading.
4) Reducing inflammatory responses: nutrition, physical exercise, emotional balance, minimal stress, allergies' control, refined sugars, insufficient Omega 3's, excess of Omega 6's, growth hormones present in meat/non-organic dairy products.
5) Stress blocks NK cells so that the NK cells remain passively glued to the walls of blood vessels rather than attacking viruses or abnormal precursor cancer cells.
6) Stress releases noradrenalin and cortisol hormones. These open doors for nasty forces.

There are some foods that provide 3 in 1 benefits:

1) Reduce inflammation
2) Stimulate the immune system and
3) Protect against free radicals

Such foods include apples, beetroot, blueberries, Brazil nuts, mushrooms, olive oil and pumpkin seeds.

Important: Nuts **do not** contain any Vitamin B. This vitamin is vital for wellbeing…

B6 – For white blood cells (bananas, cabbage, peppers, beef, liver, kidneys, wheatgerm)

B9 – Highly effective in preventing breast cancer

B12 – Cell division and growth (sardines, egg, cheese, mushrooms, pork, beef, kidneys)

Nuts are vital to include in your diet. Below are examples of which nuts are 'the king' for different health benefits:

• Iron	• Cashews
• Fibre	• Almonds (for calcium)
• Omega 3	• Walnuts
• Selenium	• Brazil nuts
• Sterols	• Pistachio (for iron)
• Vitamin E	• Almonds

Seeds are also vital to include in your diet. Aim for less Omega 6 and more Omega 3 as too much Omega 6 can stimulate cancer growth/inflammation; so limit sesame or sunflower seeds!

5. Acidity in the Body

Acidity is another major commander in the nasty army and so reducing acidity in the body is essential.

1)   The pH scale is the scale for measuring acidity and alkalinity. The pH scale is from 1–14. Less than seven is acid, more than seven is alkaline.

2)   The human body should be slightly alkaline, approximately 7.2-7.4 pH.

3)   The immune system works best when slightly alkaline!

4)   Water has a neutral reading of approximately 7 pH.

5)   A daily quarter teaspoon of sodium bicarbonate in lukewarm water is helpful in developing an alkaline body.

6)   Salt (sodium) poisons your cells; it increases cellular acidity and sets up the conditions that breed cancer.

7)   The inside of a cancer tumour is **very acidic** – pH 6.2

8)   High sodium foods are potentially 'acid cell' makers.

9)   Potassium and magnesium foods are potentially 'alkaline cell' makers, so they are 'good' to include in your diet. Aim for 5x more potassium than sodium.

10)   Cheese is the **most acid** generating food of all!

11)   Processed meats, dairy foods and egg contain high amounts of the acids that must be eliminated or reduced by the body.

12)   Nuts, seeds and vegetables contain alkaline minerals which help to balance high acid levels in foods which contain protein, e.g., meat, dairy foods and eggs.

13)   Fruits and vegetables also contain acids but they are in a form that is easier for the body to dispose of.

14)   The body uses up valuable nutrients in order to get rid of undesirable acids.

15)   The liver and kidneys become overworked in trying to remove acids from the body.

16)   The liver can also become overloaded neutralising the lactic acid produced by cancer cells; as well as dealing with bacteria, parasite, viruses and drugs.

17)   Examples of acid producers also include stress, lack of sleep, alcohol and cigarettes.

18) Acid bodies spread cancer.

19) Examples of alkaline products also include sunshine, soya, whole brown rice, dried figs, raisins, and wholefoods.

6. Digestion, Absorption and Guts...

A healthy gut is an ally to be reckoned with.

- Turn your dinner-plate into a rainbow of colours; different colours often indicate different compounds so that you are more likely be eating a healthy combination of foods.
- Focus on *when* you eat, *what* you eat and *how much* you eat! Aim for 5-6 small meals daily and eat meat/fish only three or four times a week.
- The body is made up of 75-100 trillion cells. Each cell gets 'something' from all the nutrients in what we eat!
- Each cell has more than one billion biochemical reactions per second. Food is involved in all these reactions!
- Whatever type of protein you eat, the body will break it down in the digestive tract.
- The body will use it to rebuild what it needs in the blood.
- Gut bacteria control approximately 85% of the immune system.
- Chew food thoroughly as these releases an enzyme in the saliva (ptyalin) which is crucial to proper digestion.
- Avoid diluting the body's digestive juices, either drink 45-60 minutes *before* your meal or 90-120 minutes *after* your meal; this helps digestive enzymes to work fully.
- Digested food (known as chyme) moves rapidly through the small intestine while it is being absorbed.
- The *small* intestine is approximately 21 feet x 1 inch. It has three parts: duodenum where most *digestion* occurs and the jejunum and ileum where most *absorption* occurs.
- Food can spend from 1-6 hours (average two hours) in the small intestine before it's emptied into the *large* intestine.
- The large intestine is approximately 5 feet x 2.5 inches.
- The journey through the large intestine takes approximately 14 hours.
- Carbohydrates need an alkaline environment for maximum efficiency and to be able to clear the stomach in approximately one hour.
- Protein requires an acid environment. It requires approximately 90 minutes to clear the stomach.

- The digestive system isn't designed for the simultaneous consumption or carbohydrates and proteins. So, it can take up to eight hours to pass through.

Under normal conditions, 800 types of bacteria live in the gut; 7 trillion cells and 25,000 genes! There is a microbe population in our intestines; the world of 'microbiome'. This world makes up between1-3% of our body weight. The body needs 'friendly' bacteria! A healthy gut…

1) Reduces inflammation
2) Kills cancer helps
3) Helps excrete toxins, chemicals and hormones
4) To communicate with the brain

Each night, the beneficial bacteria in the gut can 'eat' up to 2.2 pounds of yeast, moulds and microbes. Some of the neurotransmitters (chemicals in the brain) are produced by our microbiome.

- Drugs, poor eating habits and medicines kill off the good bacteria.
- Candida is a fungal colony which greatly reduces oxygen levels. Like cancer, it **doesn't** need oxygen to survive.
- Yeast invaders and fungal infections produce alcohol from their favourite food sugar!
- Acidophilus, lactic acid bacteria and bifid bacterium all help to put back good bacteria.
- Garlic, oregano, fennel, cinnamon, nutmeg, chilli and bee propolis kill off excess yeasts and microbes.

A simple fibrous diet of nuts, seeds, olive oil, grilled meats and fish and sugar free, dairy-free foods are important.

Beetroot – increases the cells' uptake of oxygen by up to 400%

Broccoli – requires a fat eaten alongside it to maximise use of Vitamin A and Vitamin K (e.g. plain yoghurt)

Pineapple – contains the enzyme bromelain. This enzyme helps digestion and the breakdown of protein.

7. The Brain

- The brain makes up 2% of our body weight and is approximately 60-70% fat.
- The brain uses 20% of all the oxygen/energy in our bodies.
- The brain uses approximately 75% of **all** the glucose that circulates in the blood and so is absolutely dependent on a stable supply of blood sugar.
- The brain needs an essential fatty acid (EFA) to facilitate the communication between the neurons and repair any damage. Fats such as Omega 3.
- When we exercise, we increase our heart rate which is vital, as this pumps more oxygen into our brain.
- More oxygen through exercise also reduces inflammation and stimulates the production of chemicals that maintain the brain's health and survival.
- The human adult brain weighs about three pounds.
- The size of an adult man's brain is approximately 10% bigger than a woman's.
- The brain has three main parts, four lobes and two hemispheres.
- The brain's three main parts are the midbrain, hindbrain and forebrain.
- The midbrain and hindbrain makes up the brainstem. They connect the forebrain to the spinal cord.
- The forebrain contains the cerebrum which is divided into four lobes.
- The four lobes are the frontal lobe, the parietal lobe, the occipital lobe and the temporal lobe.
- The brain's two hemispheres have different functions.
- The *left* side deals with thinking that is related to logic, detail, verbal…
- The *right*-side deals with thinking that is related to emotion, visual, creative.
- The brain has electrical and chemical activity all the time.
- The brain has between 86-100 billion nerve cells which are called neurons.
- Neurotransmitters are the 'chemical messengers' that help each neuron's electrical impulse 'connect' to the next one.
- Neurotransmitters regulate our moods whilst our foods affect the regulation of our neurotransmitters.

- The gut communicates directly with our brain via the vagus nerve.
- Each neuron passes on information to other neurons and can make between 1,000 and 10,000 connections (called synapses).
- There are two types of neurons – sensory and motor.
- The human brain's structure is 'plastic'. This 'elasticity' means that the brain is able to adapt to change! The brain is always changing a result of genes, culture, ageing, sleep deprivation, nutrition etc. Therefore, everything you do to keep yourself healthy also helps your brain!

8. The Vagus Nerve

The vagus nerve is a very important nerve that runs from the abdomen to the brain with connections to all the vital organs: brain, liver, kidneys, heart and lungs. It's like a sensory part that impacts on how you feel. Treat it good and it will treat your vitals good! A healthy vagus nerve is a healthy body.

Ways to stimulate the vagus nerve include:

Laughter, singing, humming, prayer, massage, cold water washing the body, exercise, no anxiety, no worries, and social interaction.

Foods that help the vagus nerve function well include: Avocado, beetroots, beans, cooked tomatoes, salmon, magnesium, potassium and yoghurt.

Like all other problems, the ways to deflate a happy vagus nerve and to negatively affect our vital organs include: Anxiety, negativity, bad diet, worry, bad habits.

Our thoughts create our reality. We can believe them and become stuck in the past with memories and fears.

We can become trapped by our fears and stuck about the future.

The only 'time' that really exists is this moment now! The **Present** moment – now – is really a gift or a present for us all.

Thousands and thousands of writers, philosophers, researchers throughout thousands of years have recognised that the mind and our thoughts are what really control us.

The more each person learns how to deal with their thoughts, the more they are able to deal kindly and wisely with all that they say and do. This helps them as well as those around them.

9. Ageing

- The human body has approximately 80 different organs including skin, heart, lungs, kidneys and liver.
- Age-related conditions are the greatest cause of death worldwide.
- The human body has 40 trillion cells.
- Hundreds of billions of cells die every day.
- The body constantly replaces dead cells.
- In old age, chronic inflammation can fuel the ageing process and so it's important to be aware of what you can do to reduce/limit stress.
- As the immune system ages, it becomes weaker.
- An ageing immune system can respond weakly to things such as vaccines.

Things to help the ageing process include:

- Learning about different lifestyle methods
- Making choices to limit potential age-related problems.
- Reducing stress – stress dampens the immune system, so the body becomes weak.
- Positive thinking – this lowers levels of the stress hormone called cortisol.
- Cortisol – released when stressed – accelerates the ageing process of the brain.
- Establishing good quality and regular sleep patterns
- Drinking water regularly – hydration
- Exercise – benefits are plentiful including helping metabolism, bones, nerves, circulation etc.
- Diet/nutrition – limiting sugar, alcohol.
- Understanding how to keep the gut flora/microbiome in the body healthy.
- Reaching and maintaining a healthy body weight. Being aware that the 'fat' we cannot see – called visceral fat – is the most dangerous. It is the fat deposits (adipose tissues) deep inside our bodies.
- Limited alcohol
- No smoking/drugs

- Keeping teeth clean to avoid decay, inflammation etc.
- Keeping eyes healthy – exercises, regular check-ups, avoiding polluted areas etc.

The body has little 'energy generators/batteries' called mitochondria. These help the cells in the body work well. Exercised muscle contains more and better mitochondria than sedentary muscle. As we get older, the body has less of these which is one reason why the brain, heart and muscles get weaker. They need a lot of energy to work well!

10. Cancer

Cancer is one of the main diseases in our society. Main causes are diet, stress, lifestyle, pollution and a diet with high glycaemic (GI) foods. All of these will contribute to the onset and growth of the disease.

It is vital to also eliminate ultra-processed foods as well as reducing/limiting the following:

Sugar-containing beverages: Sodas, sweet tea, sports drinks

Processed foods: bacon, sausages, ham, corn chips, pretzels and so on

Fast foods: burgers, fried chicken, pizza

Bakery/grains: Doughnuts, white bread, cakes, biscuits, cereals (unless wholegrain)

Potatoes: Mashed potatoes, French fries

GI foods

High levels of GI foods raise insulin levels which causes inflammation. Inflammation helps sustain growth of tumours. If the tumour's environment is deprived of inflammatory factors needed for its growth, the tumour will **not** succeed in spreading. Therefore, aim for low GI foods. These help to regulate blood sugar levels which, in turn, reduces insulin secretion which, in turn, reduces the growth of cancer cells.

Low GI foods include

- Apples – Green apples have less sugar than red apples (approximately one teaspoon less)
- Beans
- Beetroots
- Berries: raspberries, blueberries, strawberries – contain more Vitamin C than oranges Blackcurrants (weight for weight four times more than oranges)
- Carrots (contain chromium which can help stabilise blood sugar levels)
- Cherries
- Grains such as quinoa, bulgur and buckwheat.
- Kiwis (one kiwi has more Vitamin C than one orange)
- Lentils and pulses (also provide valuable protein) Oats

- Pasta
- Pomegranate juice
- Rice
- Unrefined foods

Stress

Stress is not good news for any ailment and can help in the development and growth of many diseases. Stress releases a hormone called cortisol. Cortisol causes increases in blood sugar, cholesterol and the dreaded inflammatory process. Cancer loves inflammation as it helps it grow.

Lifestyle

It goes without saying really…things such as smoking, drug abuse, pollution, poor diet are just a few examples of **friends** of cancer. **Lack** of exercise is also a friend to cancer. Lack of exercise is also a friend to cancer because exercise promotes a good intake of oxygen. A prime enemy to the disease.

Here's an army on standby

Slowing down tumour growth	Cutting supply of blood to tumours (angiogenesis) to reduce tumours from spreading	Inflammation reducing	Forcing cancer cells to die apoptosis	Stimulating the immune system	Anti-oxidants to protect against free radicals
Chocolate (Dark more than 70% cocoa)	Apples	Apples	Berries: Blueberrie, Cranberries	Beetroot	Beetroot
Fruits and vegetables (colourful /organic)	Beetroot	Beetroot	Chocolate (Dark-more than 70% cocoa)	Brazil nuts	Berries: Blueberries, Strawberries
Lentils & pulses	Broccoli, Brussel sprouts, Cabbage, Cauliflower, Spinach	Citrus Fruits: e.g. Oranges, Grapefruit, lemons, tangerines	Garlic (single best anti-cancer veg), Onions, Chives, leeks	Fruit & vegetables (Colourful/ organic)	Chocolate (Dark-more than 70% cocoa)
Mushrooms	Celery	Ginger		Grapes/grape juice (dark red)	Fruit: Cherries, Mangoes, Kiwis, Peaches, Watermelon
Nuts: Walnuts, Pecans, Hazelnuts	Garlic	Grapes (dark)		Mushrooms	Ginger
	Green tea (steep for approx. 10 minutes)	Green tea (steep for approx. 10 minutes)		Pumpkin seeds	Green tea (steep for approx. 10 minutes)
	Linseeds	Nuts: Almonds, walnuts		Shellfish	Nuts: Brazil nuts, Pine nuts, Pecans
	Herbs: Basil, Mint, Oregano, Rosemary, Thyme	Oily fish: Herring, Mackerel, Salmon		Tomatoes (lycopene)	Oats
	Olive Oil	Olive Oil			Oily fish: sardines, salmon
	Parsley	Pomegranate Juice			Olive Oil
	Tumeric (most natural anti-inflammatory to date) Add it to stews bolognaise and Salad dressings	Seeds: Linseeds, pumpkin seeds			Seeds: Pumpkin seeds, Sesame seeds and Sunflower seeds
		Turmeric			Sultanas
					Vegetables: Avocadoes, Carrots, Mushrooms, Onions, Red & Orange Peppers, Red Cabbage, Spinach, Tomatoes, Watercress

11. The Heart

The heart is one area which I have a lot of personal experience in, as you will have read about here in this book. The biggest killer in our world: Heart Disease.

This vital important organ pumps blood around our bodies. It carries oxygen where it is needed to all other body parts and other vital organs, keeping us alive and kicking. Just like the boiler in your home is the central pump circulating heat and hot water, so is the heart pump the centre in our bodies circulating blood (oxygen). The only difference is that if the boiler stops working you have neither heat nor hot water. You still have cold water although you may smell a bit due to lack of washing. If the heart stops however, so do **you**!

In order for the boiler and the heart to pump efficiently, they have to have water and blood coming in first respectively. Free flow therefore is crucial. A must! It is similar to your local shop; constantly bringing in supplies for you to buy so that you can eat and drink. If the shop closes down and there is no supply, you don't eat or drink. I know you can say well, I will find another shop, yes, that is true. With the heart however, there is only one. If there is no supply, there is no you. So, the pathways (main arteries) in and out of our heart must be kept clear.

We are born and carry on living our lives, assuming all is well. And why not? The problem is that most of the time we do not have a clear sign to think otherwise. Or do we? Some people are born with a hereditary heart condition called Familial Hypercholesterolemia (FH) and don't know it. Close blood relatives with heart disease can make you more likely to get heart disease, finding and treating this condition early therefore reduces coronary heart disease risk by 80%. Other people, through lifestyle, can have heart disease and don't know it. This is either because they believe they are fit and young and it is not something that will happen to them and therefore ignore little signs, or there might not be any obvious signs; that is also possible.

These two categories of people unfortunately have heart attacks. People whom we hear about in the news, who were very often reasonably fit or fitter than most, and so this comes as a total surprise to everyone. Many people do know they have heart problems and take all kinds of medication. Some also have serious operations but, there are those people, who are surprised when they suddenly have heart problems. People who might have ignored little signs, however slight they may have been; like my little ache in the shoulder or they had no gauge to indicate otherwise that something wasn't quite right.

This is where regular exercise comes in and that is how I knew I had a problem. Exercise is a great way to help keep your heart healthy and, just as important, it provides you with a gauge that tells you, directs you to something that was not there before. If you exercise regularly, you get to know what is normal and good and when all is well. When something pops up that is new, like an ache or pain, fatigue or breathlessness for example, you monitor this straight away and, depending on how long it goes on for, or its severity, you immediately know that you need to seek medical advice. *If in doubt, check it out! A*s I did with my little ache in the shoulder. It was not in my shoulder on the heart side but on the right-hand side. So you can see, how a lot of people would have just ignored the pain as it was not close to the heart. I say if it is anywhere above the belly button, just see to it! I was told that it was almost a certainty that, if I had ignored the 'little ache', I would probably have had a heart attack and, even worse, not be here writing this for your protection. I am happy that I am though!

You will almost get a clear sign that something is not right through exercising, in addition to all the wonderful other benefits associated with exercise. Healthy people who do not have an exercise gauge, watch out for those obvious symptoms described; slight although they may be and check them out. This is also important if you are aware of relatives who have had heart disease in the past, and so do check and eliminate the risks associated with the hereditary Familial Hypercholesterolemia disease.

As with all the other good stuff mentioned in this chapter, the heart benefits from most healthy alternatives with particular emphasis on the following:

Exercise – The heart's number one friend and ally.

Good hydration.

Good diet – eliminating saturated fats found in lamb and processed meats. Go for lean meats such as 95% lean ground beef or pork, tenderloin or skinless chicken or turkey.

Reduce sugar and refined carbohydrates such as cakes and biscuits.

Include nuts, seeds, and soya products (tofu).

Include legumes such as kidney beans, lentils, chickpeas, black eyed peas and lima beans.

Include fish, oats, berries, tomatoes, fruit and vegetables.

Look after your heart! Keep the shop open!

Chapter 8
That's Life!

Living in Folkestone, so far, has been truly wonderful. It is Monday, August Bank Holiday 2022 today. The Carnival is back on the streets of Notting Hill and outside my old front door after two years in exile due to the Covid pandemic. I was living there when the first Carnival happened, there when the Riots happened, and I have some great and not so great stories and memories. Sounds like another book is emerging! The sun is shining so I may go for a walk down by the Mermaid Beach or The Leas or a trip down to nearby Dymchurch. I sincerely hope this book was enjoyable and informative to read and will help you choose routes you want to follow.

I have not freely used words such as: "You will be cured, you will have freedom from" or "you will beat," because when it comes to wellness and depression, I do not believe these words apply. You can contain, yes! You can control, yes! You can be free from, yes! You can stay on top of, yes!

You cannot be cured, have freedom from, beat depression and some other serious illnesses in the true sense of the word. Terrorism, despots, hunger, injustice…Have we cured, beaten, have freedom from? No! In addition to all of these problems, what about these scenarios. We are walking in the countryside or some beautiful beach and yes, there it is. Empty beer cans thrown aside, half-eaten food and take-away cartons everywhere. Why? Have we beaten, cured, had freedom from this social problem? No! It's a bit like a song I perform entitled *That's Life* by Frank Sinatra.

"That's life, that's what all the people say, you're riding high in April, shot down in May, but I know I'm going to change that tune, when I'm back on top, back on top in June".

*(especially when I dip into my H.A.H.A.). "I said, that's life and, as funny as it may seem, (not really funny), some people get their kicks **stomping on your dreams**."*

Are you familiar with these types of people? They are everywhere. Just like depression, terrorism, despots, hunger and injustice. There are many aspects and situations that lead to the formation of these groups and events. Terrorism equals religious differences, hatred and ignorance. Despots equals greed and power. Injustice equals negligence and corruption. Hunger equals greed, corruption and negligence. Depression equals moronic actions, people who get their kicks stomping on your dreams, unfair results, morons who litter our streets, our minds and by being let down by the big players in our society.

We have to rise above all of these. Acceptance is a good deposit for the H.A.H.A. because these people and their actions are part of our world and, it seems, they are here to stay. Another good deposit is to go out there with one of those contraptions that help pick up litter and do your bit. If you can't beat it, at least stay ahead of it.

It is the same with serious illness like cancer and heart disease. You can avoid being affected by it and stop it from killing you, but cured, freedom from, beaten it. I don't think so! Because in order to maintain and stay healthy, you have to carry on with the regime that stopped it in the first place. You have to have control! My wife and I are often told: "Well done, you have beaten cancer."

I wish that were true. We say thank you but we know that is not the case. We are free from it and hope that it will always be the case forever, but we know, as most people do, cancer and heart problems can re-occur when you least expect it. A fact!

I got to write this book by circumstances; certainly not planned. I enjoyed doing it, although some parts evoked having to re-live sad times, which I found to be very upsetting. But I guess that is the price any writer has to pay by writing true events.

I hope it helps you to some degree. H.A.H.A. works because it is not a perfect world. You have to help make it a perfect world, or, at least, believe you can for yourself and others.

Chapter 9
Anti-Depressants (2)

Wo! Hold the phone! Hold the phone! It's 7:15 pm on Tuesday 30 August 2022. I am about to dive into the bath and soak my weary bones when my wife calls out: "Hey, did you read this article about depression in *The Daily Mail* today?" WHAT? NO! I did look at the paper but obviously must have missed that one. I immediately had this thought that someone had stolen bits from my unfinished manuscript, and it leaked out. Some mind I have! I had to check it out though in case it was true. Did I really think that? True, I did. So, half naked, I rushed to have a glimpse at this article before I got into my bathtub. Phew! It had nothing to do with my valuable unfinished manuscript. But more to do with a newly produced anti-depressant pill. Here we go again! I went for my bath and will read about it later. Am I ever going to finish this book?

The new wonder drug hailed as a game-changer and approved in the US is called Auvelity. Apparently the makers are very happy as the shares in their company have risen by 40% in just one day. The research shows it rapidly reduces symptoms within a week, with some patients experiencing remission. In other words, no symptoms at all by week two. No wonder the shares shot up by 40%. Other drugs apparently take about eight weeks to show any positive effect. The twice daily pill works in a completely different way from current ones in all its makeup. The claim is that it prompts the brain to form new neural connections, allowing for more **positive thought pathways** to develop. Positive thought pathways! Wow! Isn't that positive thinking? I bet you get one of those by simply handing a couple of pound coins to some hungry person in the street or going for a nice brisk walk. More good news though. This drug apparently does not have the same horrible side-effects as old anti-depressants such as sexual dysfunction (reported in over 70% of patients in one 2016 study), withdrawal symptoms and weight gain as well as feeling emotionally numb. Up until now, I was not aware of these side-effects from current anti-depressants. I knew it was not good news but now I am wiser thanks to this article. WHAT! These side-effects are enough to double your depression than cure you. Emotionally numb! WOW! What the hell is that? And sexual dysfunction! Wow!

Never fear, however, this new wonder drug does not have these awful side effects, oh no, just a few of the most common ones. Dizziness, nausea, headaches, sleepiness and dry mouth, oh! That's alright then! Are you serious? These side effects are enough symptoms to keep some people in depression forever.

Chapter 10
Statins

There was another article in the same newspaper – *Daily Mail* – on the same day, 20 August 2022. I missed that one as well. Strange! Two topics coming up together on the same day on the same subject that I am just writing about. The second article was written by Shaun Wooter (health correspondent). The title was: 'Statins don't lead to aches and pains; landmark study finds side effects are just old age'.

If you go back to what I had to say about statins in 'Chapter 5, Medication – Friend or Foe' you will note that I believe statins work, no doubt about it. I did not say the drug causes aches and pains. What I did say was that statins heighten pre-existing aches and pains people already had; making these problems even worse. In my case, I suffer from aura migraine sometimes, the occasional headache, the usual knee pains and, of course, the mandatory aches and pains associated with later years of life. In my experience, these problems were heightened by about 20% by taking statins for four years non-stop. As someone who was taking statins, I mentioned these facts many times to consultants at lipid clinics in London Hospitals and now in Folkestone. Nobody ever disagreed with me on the fact or that I found statins heighten depression, as well as probably also having something to do with causing it.

I would recommend that a study is carried out based on whether statins heighten these ailments and cause depression and stop this ongoing outdated question on causes of aches and pains. It is very obvious that elderly people have these problems and it is also obvious to me that statins do heighten the pains by about 20% and contribute to depression by about 11% as I have discovered through doing my own research. For me, I had a choice to watch my diet especially since I had stents' implants and to use natural methods to keep my cholesterol steady and to lower it to an acceptable level. Taking statins was not a pleasant experience and I still do believe statins increase levels of depression as mentioned.

I think I will keep away from newspapers for a while. Well, at least until I finish writing this book. I do hope it has been helpful to you and, please note, it is the experience of a couple of people wanting to pass on factual knowledge and choices they have made. Check everything, question everything; especially if it involves your one and only wonderful life. H.A.H.A. will help.

Chapter 11
The Real

Today is Tuesday 8 September 2022. I started writing this book in March 2022. By sheer coincidence, my brother-in-law Costas passed on in May and my beloved mother in June. I am writing about depression and here I am right in the middle of one of the main causes. Sadness does not get any worse than these moments.

Today, as I am sitting here trying to continue with my story at 13:41 and having just written 'these moments', I get a telephone call from my sister's daughter informing me that my sister Thelma, whom I told you about in previous pages 'Chapter 3, Depression from Illness', the one who always said: "I have one life to live and so I will enjoy it," had passed on. I actually spoke to her yesterday when she called me for a chat, sounding ill. We always called each other regularly. I always kept a clear channel open for her because of her depression and ill health as someone who was always there for her and, I always was.

I told her I was writing about her in my book as the person who said: "I have one life to live and so I will enjoy it."

She said, "And the one that did not listen."

Laughing I said, "Yes that one" and was happy I was writing about her, laughing some more.

I told her, "I love you" and that was the last time I spoke to my little sister Thelma.

She was 72 years old. As tears are streaming down my face and probably about to break down, I am going to stop now and do what I have to do – 14:00.

It is now 16:00 and I am just walking around the flat. Bemused. Is this really happening? Have I lost three members of my family in the space of a few months in the same year? It is true. I have lit a candle again. I am alone. My wife has gone to London as she helps to look after her frail mother and stays the night. I would normally get in my car and drive to London to be with my family but, heavy rain and thunderstorms are predicted, so I will not be driving on the motorways with that lot happening. There is option two; going by train, which will take about two hours door-to-door, but, again, with this weather and crowds of people, with the way I feel! I don't think so! I decided to just sit here and continue writing as I was doing before the news of my sister! Actually feels calming in-between the tears.

I had a good relationship with my little sister. I always looked out for her; being younger and always getting into trouble. I called her a nutcase; she just laughed. She had been ill for as long as I care to remember, heart bypasses, you name it and still continued to smoke. I think that a lot of people would have walked away for many reasons, but for me, she was my nutcase and needed me. I will miss her terribly but I am happy her pain and suffering is over and so pleased I told her "I love you" before she left. Be seeing you, T!

I also had a good relationship with my brother-in-law Costas who was 83 when he passed on. A drinker and smoker and another one who could not be told how to live his life. We did not see eye-to-eye on some occasions but was always respectful, kind and generous to him. The little building repairs I did in his house, filling in forms for him and so on were greatly appreciated. Even when he was in hospital I did a little plastering repair in his kitchen as he had asked me weeks before. Someone face-timed him on WhatsApp and so I was able to show him the completed work; trying to encourage him to get better and come home. I got the 'thumbs up' and I knew; he knew that I would continue to be there for his wife; my other sister, Olive.

Unlike my father, who passed away at the age of 62, sad though it was, my lovely mother Theano who was 97 years old when her time came suffered a setback. Living with my sister and Costas, she was very upset when he passed away; more than anybody would have thought or expected. Understandable though, when you think they were all living together for 55 years. I think that was the turning point for my mother. "I believe that we all 'die a little' when a loved one goes and I think that 'little' was all my mother had left at her time of life. It was noticeable. I always maintained that whoever went first – my mother or my sister Thelma – the other would follow soon after. I was right. Thelma; who adored our mother, did leave two and half months later and, I guess, that 'little dying' was all she had left."

It does not get any bigger than the loss of a mother. For years, I was dreading the moment. I think most people do. It is a turning point for all of us especially if one is as close as I was; her banker, doctor, chauffeur, fashion advisor; I was all those people and proud to have been. Grieving is one of the hardest things I have experienced. I have had occasions before but not as hard as the present moment, when I have lost not only some of the most important people in my life, but virtually at the same time. If I 'died a little' each time, which I do feel I have, I am going to have to rely on my H.A.H.A. for extra help. Grieving as I am, I do not feel depressed with my losses because I have enormous amounts of deposits in my H.A.H.A. to dip into, in their memory. My mother especially who I cherished and being on top of her needs – and more – helped in her reaching 97 years. A great achievement and a huge deposit.

Holding her hand wherever we went. Going for a walk at the Garden Centre; choosing plants and planting in hanging baskets. One of my favourite deposits was our weekly rendezvous at the Centre's Cafe for our cappuccino and toasted cheese sandwich where we would discuss our family affairs and world problems. I am going to miss all of that and already miss her tremendously, but I know she was tired, and, who would not be reaching 97? Truly my hero too and happy she is at rest now until we meet again. And we will meet again because there is no way love like this will ever diminish. Another reason why I do not feel depressed is because this is what happens in life. It is part of our contract; we know it is going to happen and one of the best ways to prepare for this is by being kind, respectful, generous and compassionate to all; with a H.A.H.A. which helps.

I was not there when my father passed on because I was miles away working, making money. Something I have regretted ever since. When I got to his home, he was being taken away in a green body bag; that hurt me a lot. I was not ever going to let that happen again. Being self-employed, I was able to make time for myself and the people I cared for; especially the vulnerable and elderly; that was more important for me than money, cars and houses. That is why I am not rich today! I could have been very rich being a building contractor. I could have easily become a developer and seller of buildings. I turned down many big contracts and was happy making a living, paying my bills and was there for my family. Having found the singing as well meant I had everything.

I lost three members of my family this year; even one today as I write this. I am not depressed because I have nothing to be depressed about. I was there for them when they needed me and never let them down. They loved me and I loved them which I told them regularly. Amazing deposits in my H.A.H.A. which will keep me in a good state against all that is not.

> *"By caring for the happiness of others, we find our own."*
> *PLATO.*

Farewell Theano my mother, Costas and Thelma. I think they will be happy I mentioned them in this Book and happy that I finished this; especially Thelma who passed on hours ago today and I managed to carry on…Bye, nutcase! Thanks for the love.

Saturday, 10 September 2022. Yet again I thought I had finished writing this book. When I wrote the last words on the 8th, I went out to the local shop to get a bottle of wine.

When there, the shopkeeper said, "Shame about the death ain't it?"

What! I thought how did he know about my sister?

I said, "What?"

He said, "The Queen."

He showed me the news on his phone.

I said, "You shouldn't believe what you see on the phone as most are scams."

Could this be true though? I was not convinced. When I got home and, before I poured a glass of wine, I turned on the television and was shocked at the news. Yes, our Queen Elizabeth II has passed on.

'I just cannot believe it', to coin a phrase from Victor Meldew from the television series One Foot in the Grave. What is happening here? I started writing this book in March 2022 and in six months I have lost three relatives and now the Queen of England has passed on. I am writing about depression and, here I am, right in the middle of it with one of the main causes. Prince Charles, the Prince of Wales, had earlier today been proclaimed King Charles III as I write this. God save our King! We also have a new Prime Minister (Conservative) – Liz Truss – who was elected on 5 September and who replaced Boris Johnson. In fact, the Queen performed her last duty accepting the new Prime Minister before her passing.

I was distraught when I heard the news about my sister passing on and, as I sat there watching the news about the Queen which, of course I was sad about being other peoples beloved mother, I had a huge smile on my face because it dawned on me that, my sister, who loved the Queen, actually passed on at virtually the same time and day as her. Wow! The Queen and Thelma walking together to the Gates of Heaven. Yes, knowing Thelma, yes I can believe that! I can just see it now with a smile on my face.

My sister shouting out with her London Cockney accent, "Hello, luv, what are you doing here?"

One for my H.A.H.A. definitely! I believe, knowing my sister Thelma, that the Queen could not have had a better travelling companion and, I think her Majesty would not have had it any other way either. Just like my sister. Always in the middle of things. The Big Exit. And, now, there might be a Bank Holiday on that day so no excuses for forgetting the flowers for her. We buried Thelma on 26 September. Her coffin was carried in a beautiful glass carriage by two beautiful black horses. As we followed behind, in the streets of North London the beautiful glass hearse for all to see and bringing traffic to a standstill, it made me wonder who the real Queen was.

So, how do I feel about all this? Well, writing about my actual feelings, recording these incredible events is a huge deposit for my H.A.H.A. Yes, I am grieving naturally having lost so much of my life's routine and loved ones. I have cried a lot. My eyes are swollen and there's more to come in the future. But I have not stopped the writing. I have not taken to my bed. I have carried on with my exercises. I have not put on pounds in weight nor 'taken to the bottle' I have so many good deposits in my H.A.H.A. to tap into that will counteract any danger in falling into depression. Deposits like the love for my mama and hers, being Costas's problem-solver and never abandoning my non-obedient sister who now has walked with the Queen to Heaven, these will hold me in good stead for ever…

It has been great writing this book for many reasons. One, of course, was taking out of my mind and body, the stored events; especially sad events and putting them on paper and clearing out my memory stick as they put it; clearing out files from the computer; that feels good. Another deposit for my H.A.H.A.

The most important task was to find answers; helping to heal myself from depression which was there. Having taken myself back to some important incidents in my life, I now realise that my problems started way before the anti-social episodes and the let-downs I mentioned earlier. They just 'poured fuel onto the fire' which eventually took me to West London Charing Cross Hospital. I have got a lot of answers by writing this, especially writing as the events were happening and I am going to be fine!

I really do hope you get something from this book as well or, at least, it made you smile with some of my stories.

You are wonderful, you are beautiful and don't forget it!

Can I go back to the music now? I hope so. And, you know, I think I am going to be an even better singer from now on.

George Ides – Ol' Brown Eyes is coming…

Chapter 12
Surreal the New Real (2)

Again just when I thought I had finished, current events have prompted me to carry on.

Both my parents passed on while under the care of the NHS. My father was 62 years old. He was not a health-conscious man; he smoked, drank and was a professional gambler, so someone whom you can describe as not living a healthy lifestyle. He suffered a slight aneurysm in his main artery to the heart which was caught early and was being treated for. The pain from the problem got worse one day and he was admitted into hospital. As is well known, an aneurysm can kill you instantly, so we were happy he was safe in hospital. After a couple of days and, while I was not around, as I assumed that something as serious as an aneurysm would need a lot more care and certainly a lot more days in hospital, he was sent home. As his main carer and registered as next of kin, I was not informed. That evening my father called me complaining that he still had pain in his chest. Surprised that he was home, I assured him not to worry as the hospital would not have sent him home if they thought it was serious and I would call on him in the morning. My father was found dead in the morning by my sister who went to visit him as he was living alone in a flat near her. Why would they let someone out of care with an illness that can kill you? They did and it did. I tried to fight this injustice but, unfortunately, I chose an idiot lawyer who botched things up so I had to accept the outcome. Something that has been hanging over me since. I have come to terms with this for many reasons. He was seriously ill and a person who did not look after himself and I did try to be there for him and 'fight in his corner'.

My mother passed on recently which I have written about in this Book. She was 97 years old and we – the family – were very proud and pleased that this lovely old lady had reached this age from what we and other people believe was through the care and love we gave her. I especially as I was in charge of her medical needs, her medical records, her medication...Nobody did anything without consulting me first. Once she was told to consent for an endoscopy procedure while in hospital for checkups. She phoned and told me about this and I told my mother to say no. I did not think this was necessary knowing her medical history. She told the medical team that 'my son said no procedure so no signing'.

They tried to tell her that: "Your son is not doctor and you should listen to us and your consultant."

But she said, "No speak to my son."

They never did call me, and the endoscopy did not happen. I was there at every appointment, two knee replacements, a pacemaker and a new heart valve procedure.

In June last year 2022, my mother developed a pain in her back and was vomiting. I could not be there as I had moved to Folkestone. My mother was living with my sister Olive and her husband Costas in Palmers Green, North London. My sister called me as she always did whenever there was a problem with our mother and I suggested she call an ambulance, taking into consideration her age and how long this problem had lasted. I intended to be there as soon as I could. I told her where to find mother's medical records to take with them.

While in hospital at North Middlesex, my mother was diagnosed with having gallstones and a slight infection. After a couple of days there, we were told that she needed to be taken to St Bartholomew's Hospital where they had the special Xray equipment needed to carry out the test on her gallbladder so as to ascertain the seriousness of the problem. There was a waiting list as you can expect and so they decided to keep her on medication and comfortable until there was a slot available. My mother walked into this hospital, she was able to go to the toilet and function normally. We did notice that the strong medication given to her was making her a bit dizzy and confused and so we brought this to the attention of the staff there. We also informed them that she was 97 years old and the effect that the drugs were having on her therefore meant it would be necessary to put the bed bar rails up when she was in bed, in case she fell out of bed and a close eye be kept on her. We were assured this precaution would be put in place.

A few more days went by and it became evident that the appointment at St Bartholomew's was still not going to happen soon. The consultant therefore decided that since my mother's condition was stabilising and not, in his opinion, serious, he would discharge our mother to go home with medication and wait for the appointment there. My mother and us – the family – were delighted with the news.

Sometime during that night, my mother fell out of bed as rails were not put up and there was no one there to help or respond. She was later found and taken to Xray where they found a slight fracture to her hip bone. A 97-year-old lady, heavily sedated who was able to walk and function normally was now bedbound with more drugs to compensate for the fracture on her hipbone. There was no returning from that. I knew that and felt instant depression and anxiety. As I expected, my mother passed on a few days later with hospitalised pneumonia and as stated on the death certificate 'a fracture to the hip'. This was bound to happen as it is always expected to happen; especially to older people who are sedated and bedbound. The family and I were devastated. We spent a lifetime looking after our beloved mother and this happens. We have lawyers on the case and will continue with that. This sort of behaviour should not happen and, if by following through, we can stop other people from suffering the way I and my family did, then that is good.

In reality though, God help us because, as things stand and, as a casualty doctor recently said, "Keep your elderly out of hospital."

I would like to add to that: Keep yourself and others out as well. Stay healthy mentally and physically and let's fight and hope to bring change to what has turned out to be a nightmare in our health system.

As I have mentioned before, writing is great for realisations, for getting things out of your head and wellbeing, putting the tension, stresses and other nasty factors on paper and easing life as new happenings come in. It is also a way of talking to yourself and by going on and on, at the end you find something that explains a lot. What I have found in this chapter is that you get a lot of stress from corporations who provide us with services, who frequently let us down, lie to us and so on…You can blame that on greed, cost-cutting and leaving them with more profits. What is surreal and very hard to accept is that the very people we go to for help, advice and healing are doing – in a major degree – the opposite. I was out there applauding the staff during the Pandemic. I was not applauding the people who run the NHS; far from it and it seems about right. Look at the outcome now – December 2022. Nurses on strike, ambulance teams on strike. The Health Service factor in our lives is a major problem and worrying. It should be something we trust and get comfort from knowing, if needed, for ourselves, family and friends that we are in good hands. Today we get depressed even at the thought of having anything to do with the NHS. The very people who complain about the rise in mental health problems in our society are, in fact, one of the main causers; that is a bitter pill to swallow. So, shout loud my friends. This has to be put right and **now**. As with neglecting your health leads to depression, having anything to do with the NHS is depression. Something we need to keep behind bars for ever.

It's now 11 December 2022. We have had three Prime Ministers this year.

Boris Johnson, the original who was sort of ousted. Then came Liz Truss who turned out to be a dud and was also ousted. Rishi Sunak the current Prime Minister who Liz Truss beat to become Prime Minister in the first place. SURREAL! Even more surreal is that this little performance has cost this country billions of pounds. These same people are the same we trust our lives, our business, our health to. We are in trouble!

They have literally thrown away billions of pounds…'Oh well, it's not our money. It's not coming out of our pockets. What's next on the agenda?' They still keep their jobs.

My household has seen gas and electricity bills rise by about 120% with higher food bills. The nurses will be striking on the 15 and 20 December 2022. The ambulance teams will be striking on 21st and 28th. The railway operators will be striking on 1,14,16,17 December and again on 3,4,6,7 January 2023. The Border Control will be doing the same as will the postal workers. All apparently will continue. Accordingly, **with no end in sight**. Surreal or what? This is all to do with people fighting for a better standard of living, for a slightly bigger slice of the huge cake which a few are gorging on, while most have to accept what they are given. Greed, corruption, waste, bad management, bad management, bad management.

Bad management seems to roll off the tongue very easily as the cause of these problems. I feel like crying it out as it repeats in my head. It has to be that! So who is the management? The government of course, who else? These are the people who manage the country. They are the people who wasted billions trying to decide who their next leader is going to be, who threw away billions in compensation to companies unchecked for eligibility during the pandemic. £6 billion there, £1 billion over there, £2 billion down there. Waste, waste, waste. Money that could have been used to keep the people on the front line of our society doing their jobs looking after the people who pay to be taken care of.

Surreal, surreal, surreal and yes, it is happening right now. And we are expected to just carry on as normal; no matter what. Okay. We will do that. What choices do we have? I am just happy that I have a chance to document these events as they happen and hope it may help in some way in the future. I am doing something about it! Yes! I knew there was a reason to carry on writing, yes!

If you can do something about it, go ahead. We need good, responsible management. There's an incentive!

In the last three years, we have had reason after reason to be thrown into depression. I am just outlining this and to confirm it is not your fault. It is surreal and we just have to find an answer even more surreal. Start with a H.A.H.A. As the old saying goes: 'Don't wait for inspiration, start and inspiration will find you'.

STOP PRESS… STOP PRESS…

As is the habit with me writing and having written here in this book, something comes up in the headlines that reiterates what I have been saying and, to some extent, with actual words I have used. Spooky! Check this out!

Daily Mail – Tuesday 7 December 2022. Front page headlines: *Agency leeches sucking NHS dry.* Exclusive by Miles Dilworth and Harriet Line.

I am sure you can probably find the whole article if you were really interested in some internet website but for now, I will reiterate some parts of it here.

'Middlemen are charging the NHS billions of pounds a year in fees for agency staff. The massive premium which is on top of sky-high wages paid to locum doctors and nurses, can be revealed today by a Mail audit. Campaigners called for action to stop firms gorging themselves on NHS money'.

The article carries on with information on how locums are raking in £17,000 per month and agencies making huge amounts of profits sending their staff on Caribbean holidays as rewards.

You can't really blame these agencies and the people who work within. If a carrot is hanging in front of a donkey, the donkey will move forward.

This area however is just one area haemorrhaging money from the NHS. There are cleaners, food and all kind of other suppliers with rumours about the NHS paying triple the amount for toilet paper and suchlike than wholesale.

The whole reality here – which is the hardest thing to take in – is that people are dying before their time and needlessly. I would not like to have that on my conscience if it were happening 'on my watch'. Prime ministers; especially of the last five years. Good luck with developing your H.A.H.A.

Chapter 13
The Real (2) and the Finale

It's Friday 30 December 2022; the last few days of a nightmare year for me and happy it will go. And the finale for writing for now. Writing is great. Hard work mentally as always I feel I have left something out; something that needs to be said and removed from my being. Since I am still doing it, it is obvious I did leave something out so hopefully it will come out now; free to fill vacant space with more positive, happy achievement for my H.A.H.A.

One more time.

It is *not* okay to be lied to.
It is *not* okay to be treated like an idiot.
It is *not* okay to accept bad management.
It is *not* okay to have one law for some and another for others.
It is *not* okay to accept waste.
It is not okay to be disrespectful.
It is *not* okay to reward failure.
It is *not* okay for people to die before their time.

There! Glad I got all this lot out of my head one more time. I suppose if this book does not go anywhere, at least its contents are out of me. I will be free to go forward with my music which is a lot more fun, makes me feel great and makes other people happy as well. Two of my gigs fell through this Christmas due to strikes everywhere and bad management, but I did complete one at the Burlington Hotel here in Folkestone on Christmas Day in the evening. It was great fun for me as it has been a while and, especially after the kind of year I had had. But I kept thinking about my mother's advice to charge them big money and so I did. It distracted me from missing her and the words I was singing. The audience consisted of two elderly groups; one from the Isle of Wight and the other from Colchester; mingled together amounting to about 80 people. I have never performed on Christmas Day and so it felt special, and I suppose my elderly audience did not want to be at home with their memories so decided to maybe deposit some Happy Achievements in their H.A.H.A. We had a lot of fun. I got them dancing and singing; collected my fat wages as per my mother's advice and 'job done'.

Whilst writing this, I have found out a lot of things about myself and my wife. We are both very authentic, kind, considerate, compassionate and caring people. Because I want to help and write the truth, a lot of things have become clearer than before. Why do I not have a Range Rover? My own house? Three holidays per year? And so on. Because it seems as though we have both spent most of our lives caring more about others, and so long as we had a roof over our heads, the things we need to function the way we want to, that was and is fine for us.

I could tell you so much about things we have done to confirm this but you will just have to take my word for it. So, what am I trying to say here? Why am I continuing? I guess it is because there is something else to say and I will say it at the end. Before then, I have to tell you about a situation that happened a few days ago because it is so unreal it beats surreal, just unbelievable.

A couple of days ago we drove to London to visit some of our relatives and spread a little Christmas cheer. The drive was very pleasant as there was hardly any traffic and, for once, I actually enjoyed driving which I normally don't. Since we could not check into one of those hotels spread out all over the country until 3pm, we bought our flowers and visited my mother's grave with them and actually planted some daisies in the soil; she loved daisies so I felt she would be pleased. We went to my brother-in-law's Costas, buried not too far away and left flowers on his grave too. Both are in Edmonton North London cemeteries. We then drove to my sister Thelma's grave in Finchley and left some flowers there. Wonderful happy achievement doing this, especially in the peace of the cemeteries; really felt good and I felt the gratitude of our loved ones who had passed on.

We drove to my sister Thelma's flat where her children are gathering for the festive season, Grant, Lee, Tara. There is a fourth – Mark – but he was not there as he had the flu. We spent some time there, happy times and we all tried not to get upset by the missing persons no longer with us. Now 5pm we decided to check into our hotel. It was a long day so we were tired. We intended to resume our visits tomorrow as we were staying for two days. I am writing and including this bit about our visit because what happened when we checked into our hotel was so surreal that I think you may learn from this and more importantly, I need to get it out of my head!

We drove to Edmonton, North London to our hotel, checked in and went to our room. The room was stuffy and so I went to open the window. There was one but it did not open. Wow! Panic. We are used to lots of air and light where we live. There was a sign on the door informing us not to worry as the air system in the room would supply the air and to just switch it on. I switched it on but it did not work, no air was coming through. Help! We are dealing with a major essence of life here – oxygen. While I was on a chair to check the airflow, the heavy plaster grille came off in my hand; it was not screwed or glued on. I just took it off because it could fall off and cause an injury. I went to reception and came back with the receptionist. He was horrified about the grille and took it away and also managed to get the airflow going. We asked for another room but there were no vacancies until the next morning. We endured the night with the airflow system going on; now louder than before, without the cover grille. So it seemed there was no natural air coming through, but have no fear there was the airflow machine pumping in artificial air from somewhere. As if that doesn't scare the hell out of you, now we had this machine humming away all night. Some people can handle that. Others, like me, cannot. I need natural air and no noise at all. What in God's name is going on? Is this really happening? Yes, apparently. According to an employee at this hotel, all new hotels are being built with no window opening and old ones are being updated to 'no windows opening'. So guests walk into these rooms with no air coming in or going out. To get air you need to switch this air machine on. In my case at the moment, you either breathe or sleep? No contest. Furthermore, the old saying: 'Air the room' is out the window or in this case no because the window does not open. Airing rooms in these types of hotels therefore does not happen. So when you walk into such a room, you have the smell and old breathing air left by the previous inhabitants. That explains a lot and the smell around the whole establishment of smelly feet and suchlike.

I am writing about this because I cannot get my head around it and to warn you to check before booking hotel rooms; especially if you value your health and sanity. If air is only going in, how do you get rid of old air? Used air, possibly contaminated air, flu air, Covid air? *You cannot.* Weren't we told during the pandemic to always keep windows open? Yes, I believe we were! So, how is this going to work when there are no windows to open?

You can see why I needed to get this well out of my head. This is supposed to be the future. I am now waiting for the headlines.

During the night, while having to keep the air flowing so as to stay alive, eyes burning (probably due to the stale artificial air noise from the air flow machine), kids upstairs stomping on our ceiling, I managed to get about four hours of broken sleep. At 7:30 am, I went to the reception asked for a refund for the second night. I also gave them an earful and then got the hell out from that hellhole. This experience blurred our enthusiasm to visit other relatives as planned and so we simply just drove back home to Folkestone. Absolutely surreal.

The next day I got onto the hotel chain and they will not forget me for a while! I completed reviews and sent emails in protest. Needless to say, I did get a full refund but that does not compensate for our state of mind, health and time wasted, working on that. So why this new policy? Is it because people commit suicide, get drunk and accidently fall out of windows? Okay that's fine but there's so many other ways of safeguarding against these activities. Fitting six inch in diameter air vents on windows that open and close to at least let out stale air, fitting windows that only open about six inches. These are two options. To deny any kind of natural air in and to stop stale air out is simply creating incubators for germs to thrive. Have these people learned nothing from Covid? Have local government-controlled authorities who grant permission for these buildings to be built just 'turned a blind eye' or just have not even thought about it? I fear for the answer. We will wait for the headlines, I guess.

I said there was more to say and here it is.

Look after and be kind to people, especially the elderly and children.

Be giving and kind to people who ask for help and money for food and warmth.

Be kind to animals and nature.

See the other side of people who do none of these things and don't punch them in the mouth; well not until you have tried to put them right, and maybe not even then. Buy them a book or shake their hand. Great deposits for your

H.A.H.A. which will help you keep on top of things and depression, the old enemy.

There is so much to write about, and I can see how enjoyable it can be and how people make a living from this. Having come so far, I think I could have made a scriptwriter for sitcoms or movies, or I could write about being born in Cyprus during the British Occupation and then the Turkish Invasion and coming over to England. I could write about teaching my 90-year-old mother how to use a mobile phone and how happy she was when she mastered receiving and making calls. About being asked by another elderly customer of mine to tune in her Smart TV and to explain to her what social media was. Precious moments that no money can buy, and I would not swap for anything. I have come across and met so many people during my building workdays…

The precious moments that stand out mostly were those with elderly people, because they had so much to say and so many stories to tell. Let's face it by reaching 80-90 years of age, one must have all kinds to share; stories that are both very interesting and informative. I could write a book about half a dozen of these wonderful people! I still keep in touch with those who are still around and always look forward to meeting up from time to time. Don't avoid the elderly. They are truly wonderful with so much to learn from. Thinking about this today, I take pride in helping these lovely people so that they can avoid being ripped off by unscrupulous workmen who have no respect, just pure greed. I could write volumes on some of the quotes given for work not needed. I take pride that I always charged a fair price for my work which some thought was unfair (low) and so would give me more. I take pride that my mother never had to use public transport or the ambulance transport service to get to appointments at hospitals or doctors and that I was always there by her side when needed. I take pride that I spent valuable time with my parents, aunts and uncles. One of my elderly customers who is now going on 97 years old; Walter, whom I helped move with his wife Kathy from their house in Lansdowne Road, Kensington to a home for the elderly in Willesden Green once said, "When you go, George, there would be no one to replace you."

I take great pride in that.

What about the smile you get from a toddler you have never met before? Priceless!

A dog you have never seen before making strenuous efforts to come and say 'hello' to you?

Because these are so special moments – you tend to remember them forever...

I have had my moan here.

I have had my say.

I have presented an opinion for good and sincerely hope it can be helpful in many ways.

People say – and that includes me – "That's Life and we just have to get on with it."

Fair enough. But we should not accept failure from people, especially those who carry on being rewarded for unfair and bad management. Look out for it and help stamp it out! Maybe write about it? Me? I will sing about it but mostly love songs.

Writing this has been a huge deposit for my H.A.H.A. and for my wife who has contributed so much. Whatever happens now, we are winners for many reasons. That feels good.

See you at the big Stage. Haha!

Chapter 14
Woo! Woo!

I finished at Chapter 13 and thought, *Oh my God! 13!* Unlucky for some. I am not part of 'the some' who have a problem with the number 13, but a lot of people do, so then I thought, *What if these people were to pick up my book, glance through and spot the last chapter being 13.* "Ahhhh, horror 13, must put this book back, not meant for me to read." No sale. So, *welcome to chapter 14.*

As we come to the end of the first month of our brand-new year 2023, what's happening? Well, the current daily topical headlines are:

HOW DO WE FIX THE NHS, THE RAILWAY STRIKES, THE NURSES' STRIKES, THE AMBULANCE CREW STRIKES, THE BORDER CONTROL STRIKES, THE POSTAL WORKERS' STRIKES AND THE STANDARD OF LIVING CRISIS?

Stop press! Stop press! Just came in today the 31 January 2023. 'Who additionally will walk out in tomorrow's Industrial Action?' The first Industrial Action due to happen in 10 years. CIVIL SERVANTS, who want better pay in line with inflation. TEACHERS, who want better pay, better pensions and protection from job cuts. What else? Oh yes, it was announced yesterday that THE FIRE FIGHTERS are thinking of strike action soon.

Serious reform, reform, reform. They have to stop blaming Covid and the Ukraine war. Other mind-boggling headlines on the 18 January 2023. Ready? Hang on to your hats!

'Scrap EU laws to help economy'. We left Europe years ago, Brexit still a nightmare, I would like to forget. So how come we still adhere to 4,000 of Europe's regulations? Hummm!

Hospitals ask families of patients to help on wards during strikes. Hummm!

Mini nuclear firm snubs Britain for the French. Newcleo blames political chaos for decision to build prototype across Channel. They must have heard about our three Prime Ministers in one year fiasco.

An article in the *Daily Mail*, Monday 13th of February 2023, by Tom Witherow; Senior Political Correspondent: 'FURY AT WHITEHALL STAFF'S £145 MIILLION DEBIT CARD SPLURGE' *(Fraud in my eyes)*. 'How civil servants claimed bottles of wine and gourmet meals as admin and bookkeeping expenditure'.

The article continues to list examples where this kind of behaviour took place and includes culprits such as a Prime Minister and other senior government ministers. This is just the 'tip of the iceberg' of one incident report. I will bet my shirt on the reality that this sort of abuse and fraud runs into billions. Our current Prime Minister, Mr Rishi Sunak recently said, "We can't afford to give our nurses a pay rise."

I wonder why?

Take a minute and look at these headlines above. Seriously! Seriously? Oh yes! It is real and so weirdly surreal. Aren't we supposed to be moving forward? I thought so, at least that is what I have been hearing for the last 60 years since coming over from Cyprus, from the promises of every new government elected.

"Let's take this country forward, together we can do it."

Have another look at the headlines above.

It seems once we are convinced to elect them in, the togetherness goes out the window and we are left with mostly a bunch of ego-driven, childish, blundering idiots with expense accounts, which some abuse as is clearly evident, that costs us dearly in all forms including the death of people before their time.

That definitely has to change. I would just like to say to these greedy people and all the other fraudsters and fiddlers taking funds needed to heal the sick, *you have blood on your hands, live with that!* No room for a H.A.H.A here for these sad people. 'You reap what you sow', believe in that!

Reform! Stop the waste, stop the fraud, stop rewarding failure and stop bad management. Strip out the weeds and plant new honest, sustainable fruitful seeds. Seriously! No more excuses!

And now for something completely different.

BOOK GEORGE IDES (Ol' Brown Eyes)
FOR YOUR NEXT EVENT...

Go here! www.georgeides.co.uk

I knew there was a reason for writing this book, my advertisement! After millions of copies of this book have been sold worldwide, with my advertisement in it, I could become famous, a Youtuber, sell millions of my music plays, make huge amounts of bread (money) which I can give to the welfare of the elderly, children and animals. I could even afford to buy an electric Range Rover. Second hand will do, I am okay with that. Sounds good to me and my H.A.H.A. Happy days.

www.ingramcontent.com/pod-product-compliance
Lightning Source LLC
Chambersburg PA
CBHW060422290526
45791CB00002B/847